Allergy Relief

How to Completely Cure Allergies and Feel Free Using Natural Remedies

(The Truth about Allergic Reactions, Allergy Symptoms and Allergy Relief)

Edward Suggs

Published By **Simon Dough**

Edward Suggs

Allergy Relief: How to Completely Cure Allergies and Feel Free Using Natural Remedies (The Truth about Allergic Reactions, Allergy Symptoms and Allergy Relief)

ISBN 978-1-998927-84-5

No part of this guidebook shall be reproduced in any form without permission in writing from the publisher except in the case of brief quotations embodied in critical articles or reviews.

Legal & Disclaimer

The information contained in this book is not designed to replace or take the place of any form of medicine or professional medical advice. The information in this book has been provided for educational & entertainment purposes only.

The information contained in this book has been compiled from sources deemed reliable, and it is accurate to the best of the Author's knowledge; however, the Author cannot guarantee its accuracy and validity and cannot be held liable for any errors or omissions. Changes are periodically made to this book. You must consult your doctor or get professional medical advice before using any of the suggested remedies, techniques, or information in this book.

Table Of Contents

Chapter 1: How to Determine Whether You Have Allergies

Do you recall you is probably allergic to some thing? If so, you is probably searching out affirmation. The first-rate news is that there are various steps you may use to decide whether or not or not or now not you've got an allergic reaction problem.

Finding the opinion of a licensed practitioner is likewise the most effective way to determine whether or not or now not or no longer you have got allergic reactions. Doctors are one of the maximum consistent places to get an correct diagnosis. In reality, did you understand that if you have hypersensitive reactions, you will be capable of get a prescription drug from your medical physician? And in case you aren't given a prescription, the scientific health practitioner will maximum likely deliver you with more information. This fabric can encompass herbal techniques to alleviate allergic reaction signs and symptoms and symptoms or advice about the manner to cope with them.

A series of steps might be taken in order for a healthcare enterprise to determine whether or now not you have got allergies, further to the shape of allergic reactions you have got have been given. They can ask you to head returned home and do your very own experiments, which consist of if you are allergic to pets. This approach isn't always taken, even though, so a few medical doctors are concerned with what will occur if a immoderate allergic reaction occurred. As a surrender quit result, a chain of examinations will nearly sincerely be finished underneath the supervision of your medical doctor or each different licensed professional. If you have got a meals hypersensitivity, you will be required to pattern substances which you suspect are triggering the reaction, and so on.

Another approach a health practitioner can use to make an hypersensitivity prognosis is to ask their sufferers to give an explanation for their symptoms and signs and symptoms. In truth, signs are a easy manner in order to determine whether or no longer or no longer you have got hypersensitive reactions. While some allergies have top notch symptoms and signs and symptoms and signs and symptoms, you may be aware that all of them are pretty similar. Hives, a runny cough, sneezing, lung pain, and postnasal drip are a number of the symptoms and signs. Many which might be allergic to high high-quality meals can also lose recognition or have problem respiratory. If you have got a number of the ones symptoms and signs, you could looking for clinical hobby proper away. When it includes doggy allergic reactions, the above-stated signs and signs and symptoms are not unusual, regardless of the reality that awesome people may additionally additionally increase pores and skin rashes at the equal time as their pets have rubbed up in opposition to their pores and skin.

As formerly said, meals hypersensitive reactions, especially peanut allergies and wheat allergies, are stated to motive the most immoderate allergies. If you believe you studied you have those meals allergic reactions, you need to proper away prevent consuming wheat or peanut products and are seeking out clinical hobby. However, whether or now not you have got seasonal hypersensitive reactions, puppy dander hypersensitive reactions, or mold and mildew allergic reactions, you'll be capable of manipulate the signs really. There are some blogs that listing domestic remedies and natural treatments that should feature with the bulk of hypersensitivity sufferers. Natural remedy and home remedy books in the intervening time are available each on-line and offline. In fact, written materials are to be had for the ones seeking out more guidance on allergic reactions, in conjunction with a way to control or manipulate the symptoms and signs and symptoms, similarly to the manner to cope with them.

As previously said, it could be easy for high fine people to decide whether or not or no longer or now not or no longer they have got an allergy problem. When you watched you do, for example, when you have a number of the above-referred to signs and symptoms, it is also an terrific idea to look your medical doctor.

Typical Allergy Symptoms

Do you receive as actual with you might be allergic to something? If so, you'll be looking for affirmation. Over all, a few human beings experience that if they'll be able to diagnose themselves, they do no longer want to are seeking out scientific interest. This is valid in a few times, so long as the hypersensitive reaction symptoms and signs are moderate.

When it includes determining whether or not or not or not or no longer you have allergic reactions, you need to preserve an eye constant out for commonplace hypersensitivity signs and signs and signs. This is one of the simplest techniques to decide if you could see a doctor or begin making life-style adjustments. If you need to examine approximately some of the more severe allergic reaction signs and signs and symptoms, you have got a few precise selections. It is simple to do an internet search for the most common hypersensitivity signs. A simple net are searching for for can yield lots of valid medical internet web sites. You can also discover posted clinical books on the nearest library or in several bookstores. The first-class approach, although, is to preserve reading.

According to WebMD, a terrific clinical deliver, the bulk of allergic reaction sufferers great enjoy mild to slight allergy signs and symptoms after experiencing an hypersensitivity. Mild hypersensitive reactions are characterized through signs which encompass chest strain, itchy pores and pores and pores and skin, watery eyes, and a rash. Moderate hypersensitive reactions are characterised by manner of way of itchy, watery eyes, a rash, lung congestion, an itchy sensation over plenty of the body, and trouble respiratory. While maximum moderate to mild allergic reaction signs can be dealt with at domestic without the want for a experience to the physician's workplace or the medical institution, you may are attempting to find clinical interest when you have trouble respiratory and do not need the signs to worsen.

Although intense allergies are masses less commonplace than moderate to slight signs and symptoms and signs and symptoms, they will be the most extreme. As a give up give up end result, if you have hypersensitive reactions and word that your signs and symptoms are worsening, a domestic prognosis is suitable so long as you acquire clinical hobby. This is vital in case you assume you've got a meals hypersensitive reaction, considering the reality that they will be frequently even greater extreme in terms of allergies. Swelling, trouble breaking, vomiting, diarrhea, painful cramps, dizziness, and shortage of interest are all symptoms and symptoms and signs and symptoms of excessive allergies. Death may also arise if scientific interest is not received straight away after a intense allergic reaction.

As previously stated, it is totally viable for you to analyze the signs and symptoms to determine if they'll be the manufactured from allergies. Keeping this in mind, you may also need to make an appointment with a scientific expert. This is because of the opportunity of receiving a higher prescription drug that might provide you with the greatest treatment. And if you are not provided a prescription, the scientific doctor will most possibly provide you with advice and tips. For example, he or she can prescribe an over-the-counter hypersensitive reaction remedy drug or perhaps herbal strategies of alleviation. If you have fitness care, you can see your clinical medical doctor and there can be no damage in doing so.

As a word, in case you understand you have got were given a food allergy or if you have a extreme hypersensitive reaction, you may are seeking out scientific hobby right away. Mild to mild symptoms and symptoms can be dealt with at home, so intention to prevent any triggers.

Should You See a Doctor If You Suffer from Allergies?

Can you observed you're vulnerable to allegory? Are your symptoms crucial if you do? If they're no longer, you is probably asking in case you notwithstanding the reality that must see a scientific medical doctor. Of route, there can be no risk in arranging an appointment collectively together with your doctor, but you could moreover pick out out now not to acquire this. Until you decide, weigh the blessings and downsides to receiving medical interest even as you still have mild or minimal hypersensitivity signs and symptoms.

There are a collection of advantages to finding valid sanatorium treatment every time you decided you're tormented by an allergic reaction. One of them is the capabilities and experience to that you might have get right of access to. It goes without pronouncing that professional healthcare specialists are nicely-versed in their challenge. Many have years of experience diagnosing hypersensitive reactions and supporting sufferers in finding comfort. Of path, you want to do your non-public online take a look at and check greater approximately allergies, but not some thing beats the professional opinion of a systematic health practitioner.

Another benefit of receiving clinic treatment if you don't forget you're suffering from an allergic reaction is that you can get pharmaceuticals. Even despite the fact that many physicians first-rate suggest prescribed drugs at the same time as hypersensitive reaction signs and symptoms are severe, getting the alternative stays on hand for masses people. Over-the-counter hypersensitive reaction remedy drug treatments clearly do not paintings for positive human beings. Many that be troubled by using food hypersensitive reactions, together with peanut hypersensitive reactions, might not only take medication from a physicians to alleviate their results, however they might moreover accumulate medicinal drug that could maintain their life inside the destiny.

Another advantage of travelling a expert if you understand you've got were given an hypersensitive reaction is that you need to be capable of with out troubles make an appointment. If you have got a not unusual medical doctor you be aware on a ordinary foundation, what you need to want to do is make an appointment. That being said, if you are a brand new affected man or woman, it could be extra complex for you. New patients frequently have the ultimate appointments, and others are also located on prepared lists. You need to additionally search for a awesome medical doctor. Find one which accepts your medical health insurance. Someone working towards remedy in your city have to have an opportunity hastily.

While there are various advantages to locating medical treatment at the same time as you accept as authentic with you could have an contamination, there also are a number of risks. One of those hazards is the fee. You will face heavy co-pays or deductibles if you do now not have enough health insurance. Scheduling an appointment with a professional may be luxurious if you do now not have medical medical medical insurance. Having said that, it is also surely beneficial to gather medical interest. If important, search for earnings-primarily based completely absolutely physicians or healthcare centers. They will help you in saving cash. Check to appearance in case you are eligible for wonderful country-run offerings, collectively with Medicaid. This is particularly important when you have vital allergic reaction symptoms and signs.

Another disadvantage to locating medical institution remedy even as you clearly have a few non-intense hypersensitive reaction signs is the shortage of time. It isn't always unusual understanding that scientific medical doctors do no longer usually art work the most comfortable hours. You can find out it tough to gather medical hobby in case you do now not have sufficient time or can not take time off from paintings. With this in thoughts, some hospitals have bendy hours. These hours might also furthermore consist of being open on weekends or being open past due at least one night time time each week. When you have important allergic reaction symptoms and signs, together with problem respiration, you could go to the health facility.

Finally, a few human beings are not capable of are attempting to find health facility treatment due to the reality they could treatment themselves at domestic, fearing that little can be completed. When signs and symptoms and signs are not excessive, it isn't unusual for a medical doctor to prescribe over the counter hypersensitive reaction comfort drugs. In this case, you and severa others will bear in mind a go to to the physician's workplace to be a waste of time and sources.

Chapter 2: Food Allergies

What Are the Signs and Symptoms of Food Allergy?

Do you get hives after ingesting a particular food? Do you have got trouble respiratory after eating a wonderful food? If that is the case, you will probably have a food allergic reaction. Unfortunately, for sure human beings, identifying whether or no longer or no longer they're is greater hard. When the symptoms aren't important, that is most customarily the case. Keep studying for more element to help you determine whether or not you have got a food hypersensitive reaction.

Visiting a healthcare company is one of the only techniques to find out whether or not or no longer you've got got a meals allergy. Many corporations create experiments or trials to determine which substances, if any, you are allergic to. If you observed you have a meals allergic reaction, it is probably a secure concept to look a medical doctor, as they may be able to offer you with data and guidance on creating a dietary adjustment, which can also contain fending off the meals or food inflicting the signs and symptoms. Medication additionally can be administered.

As previously mentioned, hives are a trademark which you would likely have a meals allergy. In reality, hives are one of the maximum frequent symptoms of those which have a meals allergy. Hives are smooth to find out and emerge as aware about. If you get hives, you ought to remedy them with oatmeal. Pouring a cup of bowling water over oatmeal is an incredible home remedy. After a few minutes, strain and permit to sit back earlier than dabbing on the hives with a cotton ball or rag. Although this home cure can help with the hives, you need to additionally determine out what factors are causing them.

One of the maximum commonplace symptoms of a meals hypersensitive reaction is swelling of the tongue and mouth. Unfortunately, the ones effects can motive difficulty respiratory. If you have a number of the ones signs and symptoms and signs and symptoms and symptoms, you may are searching out clinical interest right away. This is crucial when you have now not been officially recognized with a meals hypersensitivity, as you do not have any supportive medication reachable.

Many that be thru food hypersensitive reactions and function a reaction can sense lightheaded or lose reputation. If this takes place to you, it is crucial which you are attempting to find medical interest proper away. In reality, insufficient medical remedy and remedy will bring about loss of lifestyles. As a stop end result, it's far crucial to acquire hospital therapy as short as you consider you studied you've got were given have been given a food allergic reaction. As formerly said, hives are an indication which you may probably have. You need to get the assist of a scientific practitioner as quickly as feasible, earlier than your symptoms get worse.

Once you have got were given been medically diagnosed with a meals allergy, it's miles vital which you tell every body spherical you of your situation. This is especially vital in case you eat dinner at the houses of buddies or circle of relatives on a each day foundation. Those human beings may additionally want to decide what now not to put in their food as a way to make greater preparations for you. This message is also beneficial if you have a reaction. As formerly noted, the ones round you want to recognize a manner to answer accurately, whether or not or no longer or not or no longer it is through prescribing remedy or calling an ambulance.

As formerly stated, it's far critical that to procure scientific attention if you anticipate you have got a meals hypersensitive reaction.

Food Allergies That Are Common

Do you receive as actual with you might be allergic to something you ate? Do a person who's allergic to those additives? If so, you might be attempting to find extra records. Some of the most well-known food allergic reactions are said under, collectively with statistics on those allergies.

Milk is a herbal meals that causes allergic reactions in masses of people. Unfortunately, milk is a commodity that can be found in masses of food, specifically bakery products. The appropriate facts is that milk is notably easy to possibility. When baking, there are various options that may be used as an opportunity.

Concerning the products that need to be reviewed, it is vital to speak with a deli employee. Did so multiple delis use the same cheese and meat reducing machines? It is likewise essential to talk with the chefs at a eating place. Often eating places use butter to oil a barbeque or to spice some elements, consisting of steaks. Keep looking for casein on food labels as nicely. Casein is a milk product that might result in allergic reactions in high-quality people.

Eggs are every different popular food to which many human beings are allergic. The actual facts is that folks which can be allergic to eggs may additionally additionally use pretty some precise options, particularly in baking. Did you understand that yeast, oil, baking soda, and gelatin can all be applied in baking? Exact recipes may be determined online or in magazines, specifically cookbooks for people with food allergic reactions.

When it entails the food that want to be examined, the ones which can be allergic to eggs need to use vigilance when using egg replacements. Egg replacements aren't necessarily made for people who are allergic to eggs. Check to make certain that no egg whites are covered. Did you recognize that eggs are on occasion used to make the froth topping for espresso beverages? Pasta is every other famous and sudden egg deliver.

A peanut hypersensitive reaction is some other famous meals allergy that many human beings have. Peanut hypersensitive reactions, sadly, are considered to have the maximum immoderate reactions. Proceed with warning whether or not or no longer or now not you've got got a peanut allergic reaction or in case your infant has a peanut hypersensitive reaction. Any mark want to be look at.

All ought to be reviewed in terms of gadgets to be checked. It isn't always uncommon for such materials, together with peanuts, to are available in numerous types. These diverse peanut-containing types can all be produced on the identical machines. As a forestall stop end result, all marks may be check. It is specially essential to avoid chocolates and bakery products.

Fish allergic reactions are also exceptionally famous. Fish allergic reactions can seem themselves in a whole lot of techniques. Any humans are simply allergic to those styles of seafood. It is recommended which you are trying to find recommendation from a healthcare provider to decide if any unique examinations want to be achieved. If no longer, it might be more secure to eliminate all fish products to be on the steady aspect.

It is a smart issue to have a have a look at all labels to determine which devices can be prevented. Having said that, it's miles essential to workout restraint even as ingesting out. You never recognize what substances are prepared at the identical grills or inside the equal cooking regions. Did you understand that awesome salad dressings and relishes incorporate fish merchandise?

Wheat allergies are a few other common allergic reaction that many human beings have. The immoderate pleasant detail is that there are numerous substitutes that may be utilized in baking. Among the ones substitutes are rice flour and corn flour, to name some.

When it includes wheat hypersensitive reactions, the whole thing should be tested. When you look at meals labels, you may take a look at that each one of them thing out that wheat might be present. It is greater steady to prevent if that is the case. Did you understand that extraordinary ice creams include wheat? While the bulk are not, it's also an exceptional issue to observe all food labels.

Parenting Food Allergy Children: Here Are Some Suggestions

Are you a determine with a toddler who has meals allergic reactions? If so, you is probably looking for some recommendation about a manner to cope with your little one's medical hassle.

One of the first subjects you can do is inform your infant approximately their food hypersensitive reaction. This is in particular vital for preschoolers and early easy college-aged kids. It is ordinary for children of this age to replace or trade treats with their pals or classmates, but this isn't constantly wholesome. The earlier you have got were given this speak collectively along with your children, the better. Be certain to speak approximately your little one's food allergy with them more than as soon as if they are more youthful. Teach older children and young adults the way to decipher meals labels on their very personal.

In addition to talking on your kids, make sure to speak to everybody who comes into touch with him or her. Teachers, university counselors, daycare services, family, and pals' parents also are covered. When an grownup is not concerned, a vast percentage of meals reactions arise outside the circle of relatives. If you are taking your baby to visit circle of relatives or a friend, you may deliver your very very own bag of nutritious, famous snacks.

It is important to take a look at all labels even as feeding a infant with food allergic reactions at home. And if a food does now not comprise nuts or wheat, it can additionally undergo a warning that these substances can be present. If this is the case, it's miles safe to keep away from it. It is likewise essential which you take a look at the labels on the components that your toddler will consume on a regular basis. This may additionally seem to 3 dad and mom to be a waste of time, however manufacturers are stated to change their recipes and the additives they use. As a result, it is maximum applicable to be healthy in area of sorry.

When consuming collectively along side your little one a long way from domestic, which incorporates at a quick food diner, a quiet sit down-down eating place, deli, or bakery, it is continuously a smart concept to ask questions first. This is particularly huge in delis and bakeries. Are all elements produced inside the equal place? Is a separate meat cutter used for meats and cheeses in a deli? If your little one is allergic to exploit or unique dairy products, they want to be. Is it viable that such meals, along side peanuts or wheat, have been used or inadvertently positioned their way into other products?

It is also crucial which you understand the way to address a meals allergic reaction. Be sure that everybody round you and your little one is aware the way to address a food reaction. If your little one is given drugs to use in the event of an hypersensitivity, make sure the medicine continues to be with you and your infant. Send the drug to the faculty nurse or daycare agency at college or at daycare. When your teenager is journeying buddies or family, make sure to deliver the drug to the person in fee and allow them to understand at the identical time as, if ever, it has for use.

When your little one has an allergic reaction to something they ate, it's miles essential to determine whether or not or no longer or now not your toddler requires medical hobby right away. Many parents need to get medication hobby for their youngsters no matter the truth that they appear to be well. This is extra than in all likelihood, especially if the food hypersensitive reaction is extremely-modern-day or if it is the primary time you have got had an allergic reaction.

As you could see, there are pretty quite a number useful suggestions to undergo in thoughts and be aware about in case you are the parent of a infant who has a food allergic reaction, specially a peanut allergic reaction. Since maximum allergic reactions rise up while a decide is not gift, make sure to hold genuinely each person who've touch collectively collectively together with your toddler up to date.

Food Allergies: Managing and Treating Symptoms

Do you believe you've got a food allergy? If you do, you will be seeking out approaches to get help or advice at the manner to deal with your signs and symptoms. If this is the information you're searching for, you could keep analyzing.

The first waft is to discern out what you are allergic to. Visit a healthcare company if you are succesful. They will administer tests or endorse you on the way to manipulate those exams at domestic. These experiments normally encompass consuming best food to look the manner you respond to them. If you break out in hives or have an entire hypersensitive reaction, you may now recognize which meals(s) you are allergic to. If you do your very own experiments at domestic, ensure you are not doing it on my own. If you have got a severe allergy, you may have someone with you who can also get clinical interest.

It can be a whole lot much less complicated to move on if you have a evaluation of and meals or elements you're allergic to. You can, as an example, find out it less complex to deal with and control the signs and symptoms. Speaking of this, a number of the stairs you can need to take to perform this are listed under.

You need to dispose of the meals or food to which you are allergic out of your eating regimen. This is essential because of the reality some meals reactions are more excessive than others. Those with peanut allergic reactions, as an example, will die if treatment is not taken proper away or medical care is not acquired right now. You don't need to take any risks on a food allergy, in assessment to puppy hypersensitive reactions, which you might truly limit your exposure to puppies. As a result, the substance or factors to which you are allergic have to be eliminated out of your weight loss program.

As vital as it is to recognize that the food or meals to which you are allergic have to be averted, it may be tough for excessive best human beings to pay interest. While a large percent of meals allergies are gift from infancy, a few adults experience them later in existence. If you are such a people, it may be hard to be able to make the essential adjustments, however it's miles essential which you achieve this. If you want to transition in region of completely exclude out of your weight loss plan, it's miles quality to gain this below the supervision of your physician. Often, please maintain your prescription available to make certain that everybody round you apprehend what to do when you have an hypersensitive reaction.

It is therefore crucial to understand that there can be choice. For example, whether you have were given a pet milk hypersensitive reaction or a wheat hypersensitive reaction, there are a few alternatives, also called replacements, that you could use. In fact, almost any food has at the least one possibility. You need to substitute corn flour or rice flour for wheat flour. You'll likely get used to the flavor proper away, if you discover any difference at all. More info on meals alternatives may be effects located on line. You can also need to shop for hypersensitivity-first-class cookbooks or education manuals.

As a note, whether or now not or no longer you've got were given been medically recognized with a meals hypersensitive reaction, it's miles vital that you examine all food labels. To be sincere, you in no way recognize what is in any of the stuff you consume. Reading all meals labeling is essential for all meals allergies, but it's miles mainly important for wheat and peanut allergies. This are components that can be applied in hundreds of meals. Even if they are now not there, you may stumble upon a take a look at that broadcasts "would possibly encompass wheat" or "would probable include nuts." Often, if you visit a eating place, ensure to inquire approximately how the meals is served. Delis, bakeries, and consuming locations are examples of such institutions.

Chapter 3: Pet Allergies

What Are the Signs and Symptoms of a Pet Allergy?

If you think you have got got a cat allergic reaction? If you do, you'll be wondering what any of the symptoms and symptoms of a domestic dog hypersensitive reaction are. If that may be a few detail you're interested by getting to know all approximately, keep reading.

When it involves domestic dog hypersensitive reactions, it is able to be hard for certain people to determine whether or not or now not they clearly have a puppy allergy. This is because of the truth that any of the reactions that certain people suffer can be exacerbated via exclusive allergies or a completely new scientific trouble. As a give up end result, anybody who suspect they may have a pet hypersensitive reaction must searching out scientific hobby.

While the signs and symptoms of a puppy allergy can often be confused with the ones of another hypersensitivity or a few other medical situation, there are greater comparable symptoms. One of these symptoms and symptoms and symptoms and symptoms is sneezing. You may have a puppy allergy in case you continually sneeze at the same time as there are pets round, most often cats and dogs.

In addition to sneezing, those who have a runny nostril or nasal obstruction may be allergic to pets. As with sneezing, it is critical to decide if those signs and symptoms are present first-rate at the equal time as you're round dogs. This is because of the reality that the ones signs aren't high-quality associated with exquisite allergies, however they also can be wrong for a chilly. Post nasal drip is a problem this is similar to those pup hypersensitivity signs.

Another everyday symptom of a domestic canine hypersensitivity is itchy or watery eyes. You need to have a doggy allergy when you have itchy or watery eyes while you're spherical a cat, dog, or one-of-a-kind pup. Itchy or watery eyes are a symptom of pup dander, which many patients are allergic to, receives into the eyes and reason infection, especially while rubbed greater vigorously.

Another indication or symptom of a puppy allergy is a pores and skin response that resembles an eczema epidemic. In reality, the most commonplace purpose of eczema is an allergy to a reason agent. A rash is likely to arise after having direct touch with a cat or canine, specifically if you saved or pup the canine. If you've got were given were given a pores and skin rash, it is critical not to scratch, no matter how a bargain it sounds which you need to, as this will motive extra pores and pores and skin pain.

Unfortunately, people who be stricken by way of puppy hypersensitive reactions are more likely to be via bronchial bronchial asthma. When the 2 are mixed, they may purpose unpleasant and disturbing signs which incorporates breathing irritation, shortness of breath, and wheezing. If you're now not capable of advantage instant remedy from remedy, medical hobby may be required.

As previously referred to, some of the outcomes skilled through the use of the ones affected by domestic dog allergic reactions can be due to distinct complications. The appropriate information is that you must be capable of see quite effects. For eg, maximum humans have troubles and word the above-said signs and symptoms inside mins of getting into contact with a pup. This is a stable way to look whether or now not or no longer you have got have been given a doggy hypersensitive reaction other than any other allergy or possibly a common cold.

When it involves what reasons those results, the bulk of human beings are allergic to animal hazard, it is the pores and pores and skin in which an animal flakes and sheds. Having stated that, some human beings have troubles with animal feces, puppy fur, and spit. A veterinarian or a few tests achieved quite simply at home will provide you with a higher expertise of what's causing your hypersensitive reaction to a pet.

Speaking of which, it has already been said that a few people have troubles with puppy fur. That is why many pup proprietors take precautions to maintain their pup's fur brief. Of route, there is typically no danger in doing so, however frequently human beings do no longer get the consolation that they have got favored for. This is because of the fact, as formerly stated, maximum humans are allergic to domestic dog dander, this is the flaky pores and pores and skin of the domestic canine in choice to the fur.

What to Do If You Have a Dog Allergy: What Should You Do?

Are you a canine proprietor who suspects you is probably allergic for your pup? If so, you is probably seeking out recommendation. After all, there's no longer some thing worse than discovering you are allergic for your preferred domestic dog or pets.

One of the number one matters you can do is test to see when you have a domestic dog allergic reaction. Certain hypersensitive reactions or medical ailments, which incorporates the flu or the common cold, can also mimic the outcomes of a puppy allergy. Many which can be allergic to pets can make bigger a runny nose, sneezing, nasal congestion, postnasal drip, a pores and pores and skin rash, or hassle respiration. Schedule an appointment with a veterinary organisation whether or no longer you are experiencing extreme hypersensitivity signs or in case you want confirmation that you genuinely have a doggy hypersensitivity.

As about a way to treatment the domestic canine hypersensitive reactions due to your dog, you should eliminate the dog from your property. If you are not in a function or no longer capable of gain this, you may need to look if you may find out it a excellent residence. Friends or circle of relatives individuals who are capable of offer for your puppy are often appeared because the better choice. And if you need to preserve your domestic dog, there are a few things you can do to get comfort from those commonplace dog hypersensitivity symptoms and signs.

The most effective way to lessen allergic attacks because of your dog is to hold your canine or pets from your sleep. The bed room is in which we spend the most of our time. As a give up result, you have to preserve your dog or puppies a ways out of your condominium. This can lessen the quantity of vexing signs and symptoms and signs you experience. It may additionally

additionally even assist you in getting a complete night time time's sleep. In addition to the condominium, it is important to investigate different rooms in which you can spend a good sized amount of time. Consider getting the canine(s) out of the room as well.

Another smart recommendation is to not permit your canine or puppies to leap on your fixtures. This is especially crucial in case you need to relax in your sofa or in a reclining chair. You do not want puppy dander or fur on your ears. Covers can be used if vital. There are lots of cloth-style covers available. They're a extremely good evaluation to the ugly cardboard covers. With this in thoughts, whether or not you have were given material covers, ensure to easy them every few days or if excessive pup fur accumulates.

Investing in an air cleanser is a few other preference for treating a canine hypersensitive reaction at the same time as no longer having to find a brief domestic for the one which you love pup. Air purifiers act with the useful resource of manner of putting off airborne contaminants such as pup dander. It is most stable to look on-line for air purifiers which can be alleged to useful useful resource folks that be afflicted by allergic reactions. A clean internet seek would possibly yield consequences for those air purifiers. Furthermore, HEPA air filters and HEPA air purifiers are well-known for his or her incredible overall performance.

Vacuuming as speedy as possible is another way to alleviate the consequences of a canine allergic reaction. In addition to vacuuming every now and then, take a short study the vacuum cleaner you're the use of. HEPA-filter vacuum cleaners are now to be had, and they will be fairly reviewed and encouraged. In truth, some vacuum cleaners are specially designed for and acquired to pup owners. You ought to check the ones vacuum cleaners.

The measures said above are satisfactory more than one the various you can take to discover relief from hypersensitive reactions because of bodily interplay at the side of your dog. As a observe, a physician is probably inclined to prescribe you prescription drugs or offer over the counter tablets which may be in addition effective. Having said that, hold in mind that treating hypersensitive reactions, in particular pup allergies, obviously is normally far better.

Pet Allergies: What Do You Do If You're Allergic to Your Cat?

Are you a cat owner who thinks you have were given a doggy allergic reaction? If you are allergic to cats, you is probably questioning what you need to do. If you're seeking out advice, hold reading because of the fact some right hints for doggy owners who are allergic to their pets are covered under.

Examining your signs and symptoms and symptoms is one of the first topics you may do if you assume you've got a cat allergy or some puppy hypersensitive reaction. When you're spherical your cat or kittens, can you've got had been given sneezing, a runny nostril, nasal discharge, or postnasal drip? Also, do you get a pores and pores and pores and skin rash when entering contact with a few element, or do you have got were given hassle respiratory without wheezing? If this is the case, you might be allergic to cats. If that is the case, making an appointment with a healthcare practitioner might be an extraordinary concept. A veterinarian may not first-rate administer tablets for you, however they will furthermore have the functionality to help you decide whether or not or no longer or not you have got a real aversion to pets.

The high-quality way to are seeking out help is to prohibit your cat or cats from your house. Unfortunately, many puppy proprietors find out it difficult to accomplish that. You need no longer be concerned if you are unable to find out a suitable domestic on your cat or cats, alongside side with a near friend or family member. There are pretty some steps you can take to get assist.

Not cuddling together together with your doggy or cats is an terrific way to alleviate the consequences of a cat hypersensitivity. Skin rashes, together with the ones much like an eczema outbreak, can rise up in pretty some processes, like near contact with a cat. As difficult as it may be to like and recognize your animals from afar, you could want to, specifically if your hypersensitivity signs and signs and symptoms and symptoms are serious.

It is likewise advocated which you maintain your cat or cats off of your chairs, similarly to not cuddling with them. Beds, reclining seats, and couches are also examples of this. This is in particular critical if you have a dependancy of sound asleep or mendacity down in your living room furnishings. Covers are an fantastic desire. If you want to apply fabric covers, ensure to wash them each few days or every time you see a huge quantity of cat fur.

Another concept is to maintain your cat or cats from your apartment. As previously said, maintain your cat or cats faraway from your room. This will help you with getting a superb night time time time's sleep. However, just locking your cat or cats out of your location is the maximum secure way. This might be to result in comfort due to the reality the bedroom is one of the most often used rooms within the domestic; therefore, it is wherein you will be inclined to reap alleviation the maximum.

Vacuuming as quick as feasible is some specific fantastic manner to reduce the quantity of hypersensitive reactions resulting from the cat or cats. Vacuuming can help with removing any of the domestic dog fur and dander that might be determined on your own family. HEPA-clean out vacuum cleaners are mainly appeared and advocated. There are also pretty some vacuum cleaners offered in particular to puppy owners. You have to take a remarkable study those vacuum cleaners.

If you are allergic in your cat, an air cleanser can and want to be used. Air purifiers of both sorts strip in all likelihood poisonous pollution from the air. Pet dander is included on this class. If you've got a cat allergic reaction, casting off domestic dog dander from the air will offer remarkable remedy. Online, you could behavior research and discover air purifiers provided to hypersensitive reaction sufferers. Air purifiers that use HEPA technology, inclusive of vacuum cleaners, additionally accumulate the high-quality standard ordinary overall performance.

Tips on Dealing with Pet Allergies

Do you don't forget you've got a home dog hypersensitive reaction? If you do, you is probably looking for techniques to get help or recommendation at the way to address developing a puppy allergic reaction. If you're, you may preserve reading due to the truth a few beneficial guidelines are given beneath.

Although there are some steps you can take to deal with or manage puppy allergic reactions, step one is to confirm which you really have a home dog hypersensitive reaction. Consult a healthcare practitioner or do your private assessments at home or within the presence of animals. Do your conditions decorate at the same time as you aren't within the presence of a domestic canine? If that is the case, you may have a pup allergic reaction. Determining whether or no longer you've got puppy allergic reactions will prevent an entire lot of time and trouble if you do now not have one.

Whether you do have a puppy hypersensitivity, or when you have a sturdy suspicion that you do, you can talk collectively along with your medical doctor. Over-the-counter hypersensitivity remedies may be recommended via your clinical physician. Based at the situations, they're capable of even prescribe capsules. While over-the-counter and prescription drug treatments are wonderful alternatives for allergic reaction treatment, it is also crucial to apprehend that there are a number of herbal steps that you may and can take.

One of the easiest methods to address a doggy allergy is to cast off the puppy or dogs. If you do not very own a pet but experience hypersensitive reaction signs and symptoms at the identical time as travelling pals or cherished ones, rethink your choice. You may, of path, restrict it slow there or lessen your trips, but you may want to strive doing something else rather. Shopping, taking issue in brunch, or grabbing a cup of espresso are each amazing options.

If you are a domestic canine proprietor and can't bear the idea of parting from your pets, consisting of although they'll be a member of your circle of relatives, keep your domestic dog or pets from your mattress room. Most humans spend the maximum in their time in their bedrooms. The ultimate detail you want to do is be stricken by means of hypersensitive reactions even as looking for to get a proper night time time's sleep. If you're a guest in region of the puppy proprietor, request to be moved out of doors if the climate is first-rate. You can also request to be moved to a area wherein pets aren't authorized.

A first rate manner to relieve the effects of domestic dog allergic reactions is to hoover as short as feasible. If you have got got were given a cat or a doggy, you may put money into a exceptional vacuum cleaner, preferably one which makes use of HEPA generation. There also are vacuum cleaners made mainly for domestic canine proprietors. If you are allergic to pets, they is probably a suitable opportunity for you. Often include add-ons that make it smooth to do away with puppy odors from bedding and furnishings.

As previously referred to, it's miles critical to have a look at that regardless of the truth that you do not non-public a cat, you may amplify pup allergies. If you meet someone who has a cat, together with a non-public friend or member of the family, tell them about your pet allergy. They won't, of direction, do away with their pets only for you, but they will take positive measures to make their domestic a higher region for you. These precautions can also include storing their pets in a few different room or vacuuming until you arrive.

As previously mentioned, whether or now not you be with the aid of pet hypersensitive reactions or take delivery of as real with that you can, it is a amazing concept to look your health practitioner. He or she might be capable of administer drugs or offer you with a few useful advice. That being said, if you are uninsured, please try any of the smooth and much less luxurious measures mentioned above.

Will Pets Suffer from Allergies?

Humans also are the number one component that springs to thoughts as each person pay attention of allergic reactions. Allergies have an impact on hundreds of thousands of humans in the United States on my own. These hypersensitive reactions is probably because of meals, mold, mildew, or the surroundings. While people are the maximum common allergic reaction sufferers, did that pets can increase hypersensitive reactions as properly? They are capable. Dogs, mainly, are the maximum common species to be troubled with the aid of hypersensitive reactions.

Many human beings are unsure a way to act almost about identifying whether or now not or no longer or now not their canine or cat has allergies. To begin, it is vital to look for symptoms and signs and symptoms and signs and symptoms. In truth, did you recognize that some of the symptoms of pup hypersensitive reactions are same to those of humans? They honestly are. If your puppy is normally scratching, this is one of the most common signs and signs and symptoms that they've an allergy. Skin sensitivity is a few other symptom. Having said that, immoderate scratching and pores and skin pain constantly pass hand in hand.

While it within reason clean for a few pet owners to determine whether or now not their dogs have hypersensitive reactions, others are even though uncertain. If this fits you, you have to are searching for clinical interest in your dog, cat, or some first rate pup that is probably allergic to some element. A veterinarian may additionally moreover carry out a number of checks as well as examine the dog's pores and skin to determine in the event that they have allergic reactions. Until you are taking your canine to the vet, you could write down any problems you have were given or something that has given you tension. For eg, did your dog scratch himself after strolling into some weeds in the out of doors? Have you just changed their doggy food, given them a contemporary puppy toy, or given them a contemporary pup bed? If this is the case, your veterinarian must be conscious.

Chapter 4: Other Allergies

Seasonal Allergy Symptoms: How to Manage and Treat Them

Do you find out yourself depressing, coughing, or sneezing on the equal time of twelve months? If you do, you must be aware which you might be stricken by seasonal allergies. While seasonal hypersensitive reactions can occur at any time of 365 days, many human beings revel in that their signs and symptoms are worst inside the spring and fall.

There are lots of vital precautions which you could in all likelihood need to take in case you need to get consolation from your seasonal hypersensitivity signs and symptoms, or no less than manipulate them. These measures, a number of which can be currently prescribed by using using medical professionals, are summarized below in your convenience.

One of the primary subjects you could do whether you choice to control or address your seasonal hypersensitivity symptoms is to pick out out the risk elements. When you've got were given a runny nostril, stuffy nostril, cough, or lung pain, it's miles most usually due to a few element specific. Pollen, ragweed, and mold are generally blamed through way of using many. Many people count on that mildew can most effective be determined internal houses and unique structures, however mold also can be placed out of doors, particularly after rain.

Another technique for acquiring remedy from seasonal allergic reactions is to get right care. While a few humans can deal with their symptoms on their very very own, some distance others want prescription drugs or no much less than over the counter pills. This is wherein seeing a medical doctor is available in reachable, specially if your seasonal allergy signs and symptoms and signs are causing you ache or pain. As previously cited, your doctor will nearly virtually prescribe hypersensitivity remedy treatment to you, especially if she or he believes your hypersensitive reaction signs and signs are crucial enough.

If you intend to deal with your seasonal hypersensitive reactions with out seeing a physician, you can most in all likelihood inn to over-the-counter drug treatments. Until using an over-the-counter treatment, take a look at all warning labels and warnings given to you. Any over-the-counter medicinal tablets can engage with one of a kind drug treatments or purpose aspect outcomes. If you need to make sure you're searching for a healthy and powerful remedy, speak to unique seasonal hypersensitive reaction sufferers you meet, a pharmacist, or take a look at articles of over the counter drugs on-line.

In addition to the above steps, which all require using a few type of remedy, it's also crucial to be aware that many people can find out comfort from seasonal allergic reactions by way of herbal or splendid smooth steps. The Weather Channel, as an instance, is well-known for highlighting immoderate pollen levels particularly locations. They furthermore achieve this at some point of stay announces and on their internet web page. If pollen stages in your region are immoderate, it might be a outstanding concept to remain indoors or a minimum of wear a defensive mask. Another excellent advice that many humans forget about is to check out any pets you could have. Pollen and ragweed receives trapped in the fur of longhaired cats and dogs, ultimately finding its manner into your property.

As formerly stated, there are some precautions you can take to alleviate the allergic reaction symptoms and signs and signs. The appropriate statistics is that the majority of these measures are simple to carry out.

What to Do If You Have Skin Allergies

Are you allergic to a few component? If you do, your pores and pores and skin may be harmed, and in a couple of manner. Skin allergic reactions, regrettably, are one of the most distressing forms of allergic reactions to attend to. This is because the rashes that many people revel in aren't most effective unpleasant, however additionally itchy and unsightly.

One of the most often posed questions for individuals who be afflicted by pores and pores and pores and skin hypersensitive reactions is how they will get treatment. There are a few moves that may and need to be taken. One of those moves is to determine out what's causing the allergy. Do you, as an example, get a rash after doing outdoor paintings? You might also moreover have seasonal allergic reactions in case you do. Can you get a rash whilst you capture a cat? If you do, you is probably allergic to pets, amongst other topics.

If you do now not already recognize what is inflicting your pores and pores and skin to reply allergicly, you must make an appointment collectively along with your medical medical doctor. You don't have anything to lose from scheduling an appointment at the same time as you have got fitness care. This is massive due to the fact many people are bowled over to find that what they felt grow to be triggering an hypersensitivity emerge as now not the number one trigger problem. Some people are lots extra taken aback to find that they may have several triggers, collectively with best elements or additives applied in positive family gadgets, which encompass laundry detergents.

One of the primary advantages you can visit a health practitioner is that they can correctly help making a decision what you are allergic to. Of direction, you have to do your very own assessments at home, however preserve with caution. This is important in case you suspect that meals is causing your pores and pores and skin rash or allergic reaction, due to the fact your signs will worsen. That is why you must avoid doing all of your non-public allergy tests at domestic, but if you do, make sure you aren't by myself.

If you have got were given decided what is triggering the pores and skin to reply allergicly, you will be able to gain alleviation greater successfully. To begin, over the counter hypersensitive reaction prescriptions can be investigated. There also are lotions and lotions that allow you to dispose of itching and hives. When you bypass see the physician, he or she might be able to prescribe particular gadgets. If you do now not want to see a doctor, you need to have the capability to speak about with taken into consideration one in all your pharmacists with out value to get their opinion on a positive over the counter allergy treatment remedy.

It's moreover crucial to phrase that you could get treatment without the use of over-the-counter drug treatments. Oatmeal, as an instance, while blended with one cup of boiling water, allowed to chill, and then strained, can also provide remedy to those affected by hives. The water derived from the oatmeal may be achieved to the pores and skin. You can also even lessen your pores and pores and skin reactions with the useful resource of getting rid of or extensively minimizing your purpose factors. For eg, in case you cannot undergo the idea of parting collectively with your domestic canine, attempt now not touching or petting it without gloves, keeping it from your bed room, and making an investment in an air purifier.

As formerly said, there are a number of causes why you may have an allergy to your pores and skin. Regardless of the deliver, there are an entire lot of techniques you may use to benefit assist.

Chapter 5: Treatments

Ways to Get Allergy Relief on a Budget

Are you allergic to anything? If so, are you looking for charge-effective hypersensitivity remedy? If you're, you can finish studying. Listed underneath are a few clean and less highly-priced steps you ought to take to alleviate the allergy signs and symptoms.

You can see a doctor if you have extraordinary fitness care. He or she can not nice be capable of supply you with pharmaceuticals, but can also be capable of offer you with more recommendation. Other herbal and clean office work to gain relaxation can be covered in these tips. Your doctor also can discover management techniques, which include how to discover ways to deal with allergic reactions. Many which have appropriate health care moreover find out this way to be easy and price-effective.

If you do no longer have scientific medical health insurance and can't pay a doctor's appointment, you have to have a study over the counter capsules intended to offer consolation to hypersensitive reaction patients. Over-the-counter drug remedies are often frequently a great deal less high priced than acquiring a prescription with out coverage. For the fine diploma of effectiveness and remedy, you can do research on line or ask others you meet for guidelines on which over-the-counter drug treatments carry out the quality. Seeking recommendations or reading net scores and comments is an top notch manner to keep money. Of necessity, while the use of an over the counter hypersensitive reaction comfort remedy, have a look at all caution labels.

Another herbal and clean manner to get allergy remedy is to keep away from or limit your proximity to the motive of your problems. For example, if you are allergic to pets and really personal one, recall asking a friend or member of the family to care for your domestic dog. If you do now not wish to take this path, or if you are not able to discover a appropriate home to your puppy, restrict your interaction with them, specifically interior. Keep all puppies as a long manner a ways from fixtures as feasible, and maintain them out of your apartment.

Make an try to preserve the residence as clean as possible. Some human beings are allergic to mildew and excessive quantities of pollen. If you're this form of humans, cleansing your home is probably tough for you. One belief is to tidy the house as short as viable. This is an exceptional way to lessen the amount of dust in your own home. You will also want to preserve in thoughts hiring a licensed housecleaner, which isn't generally less high priced. In preserving with the problem count number of clinical help, in case you are allergic to mildew and mildew, you need to strive hiring a expert mildew remover. While it isn't always lots less steeply-priced, it's miles the handiest way to discover help, and your property's price can enhance as properly. If this price is prohibitively highly-priced, hold in thoughts minimizing the quantity of time you spend on your basement or one-of-a-kind mould-infested regions.

Green tea is each other smooth and secure way to get hypersensitivity remedy. Any teas include herbal antihistamines. This are an exceptional and fairly priced method of searching for treatment. And teas that do not include herbal antihistamines may be beneficial, as tea is known for its soothing effect. Those tormented by excessive allergy symptoms can welcome the warmth and tranquility provided.

As you are probably aware, allergic reactions are to be had lots of paperwork, and those who be stricken with the useful resource of hypersensitive reactions often enjoy a whole lot of signs and symptoms and symptoms and symptoms. Oatmeal may be used when you have hives. One cup of boiling water can be used to make oatmeal. Wait a few minutes, about thirty mins, before straining. The leftover solvent can be used to deal with hives and the scalp. It is sufficient to apply a small paper towel or cotton ball.

As you may see, there are some of low-price options for alleviating exceptional common allergy signs and symptoms.

Is Natural Allergy Relief Possible?

Are you allergic to anything? If you've got, the doctor may additionally moreover have advocated pain tablets. If not, you'll probably moreover have attempted a number of over the counter hypersensitive reaction pills and gadgets. Unfortunately, treatment does now not always assist allergic reaction patients. Many human beings are left asking whether or not there is a manner to acquire more natural recuperation with out resorting to medicine.

If you're wondering if you may get allergic reaction remedy without using pharmaceuticals or over the counter medicinal tablets, the solution is sure. In fact, you will discover that you have numerous options. Some of those alternatives are not excellent more secure than taking treatment, however they're though masses less high priced.

If you do not have meals allergies, you can use meals to get relaxation. If you have got a meals hypersensitivity, you have to discourage this method or you may have every other allergic reaction that you are attempting to avoid. That being stated, whether you be with the resource of seasonal allergic reactions, pet hypersensitive reactions, mould and mildew allergies, or different hypersensitive reactions, the ones substances may be able to provide you with comfort. These meals encompass eating lime juice mixed with lukewarm water, consuming one or bananas a day, and consuming vegetable juices.

Vitamin B5 is each unique more natural way to alleviate any of the outcomes associated with hypersensitive reactions. While many humans mistake diet dietary dietary dietary supplements for medicinal drug, they will be now not. And if you may be taking a prescription, it is going to be a good buy extra strong than many hypersensitivity pills. Most experts suggest taking one nutrients B5 complement an afternoon for 2 to three months.

Despite the reality that natural allergic reaction treatment is extra often associated with herbal treatments together with sure diets, dietary supplements, and spices, there are various precautions you can take. You have to, as an instance, distance yourself from the reason variables. For example, when you have mould and mildew hypersensitive reactions, avoid areas of your own home in which mildew or mould is present, which include your basement. If you be afflicted with the aid of dirt allergic reactions, strive using a professional cleansing company or cleansing more often, which want to reduce the amount of dirt that accumulates through the years.

As previously cited, when you have a meals hypersensitive reaction, you can keep with caution. This is due to the fact that many food allergic reactions are more vital than some sorts of hypersensitive reactions, which encompass domestic dog allergies. Many which can be allergic to peanuts will bypass into surprise and die in only a few mins. As a end result, when you have meals allergic reactions, you cannot handiest restriction your meals consumption, but additionally sincerely exclude the food or additives of which you are allergic from your weight loss plan. This is crucial to recognize when you consider that certain hypersensitive reaction patients get beaten about special allergic reactions. Many which might be allergic to dogs, for instance, do not necessarily want to find out a brand new domestic for their pets, despite the fact that they need to restriction their contact. It is essential to be aware, even though, that food hypersensitivity and puppy hypersensitive reactions aren't the identical element.

As previously noted, there are various herbal allergic reaction treatment alternatives to be had. If you're searching out greater action to take, behavior a preferred net are searching for. Try buying herbal treatment books or manuals intended to help those affected by allergies.

Foods That Could Be Beneficial to Allergy Sufferers

Are you allergic to something? If this is the case, you is probably seeking out natural methods to discover rest. The appropriate information is that you do have an entire lot of picks. Food is this kind of alternatives. Did you recognize that sure food merchandise will assist you lessen or remove fine common hypersensitivity symptoms? There are others.

Before delving into multiple the unique elements you need to devour to lessen or alleviate hypersensitive reaction signs and symptoms, it is critical to maintain in thoughts the consequences of ingesting a properly-balanced weight loss program. Your body and immune device can be in outstanding shape if you eat nutritious components. This will no longer best prevent from getting the not unusual cold, however it'll additionally assist to reduce or at the least make the allergic reaction symptoms and signs greater viable.

Lime need to be placed in the matters which you could select to eat to get consolation. Most hypersensitive reaction sufferers consider squeezing the juice of one lime or 1/2 a lime proper proper right into a cup of room temperature water through using lime. Drinking this combination on a normal basis for a month or will deliver relaxation. Some human beings do not forget including round a teaspoon of honey as properly. Honey is each other meals if you need to make you enjoy better.

Vegetable juices are also endorsed. In truth, severa studies have showed that vegetable juices can assist therapy hypersensitive reactions. Many scientific practitioners even recommend their patients to consume vegetable juice. Few juices, which include carrot juice, may be ate up on their private. Many people, despite the fact that, have had success making their personal mixed vegetable juices. Many human beings maintain in thoughts combining carrot juice with cucumber juice and beet juice.

Bananas are some different meals that many people will eat to relieve allergy signs and signs. When following this herbal meals answer, it is cautioned which you eat as a minimum one banana an afternoon for a month or , ideally . While bananas can provide remedy to the bulk of allergy sufferers, they appear to offer the most treatment to those that suffer from pores and pores and pores and skin allergies or rashes that rise up due to a minor allergic reaction.

A healthful weight loss program rich in end result and veggies is likewise advocated. As formerly said, bananas and lime are considered to offer consolation to people who be with the useful resource of a number of allergies. Apples, grapes, and carrots are some particular culmination and veggies to don't forget. Some people advocate off slowly, which include consuming one fruit or vegetable first after which along with a few issue else some days or every week later. When a quick is being used, this idea is maximum extensively made.

Although the substances cited above are in all likelihood to provide you with remedy, you ought to hold with caution. It is certainly depending on the form of hypersensitive reaction you have got. Bananas, for example, is stated above as a certainly perfect manner to address folks who revel in pores and pores and skin rashes, together with from puppy allergies. With this in mind, human beings with meals allergies may be no longer able to consume a banana without experiencing an allergic reaction. That is why, in particular in the case of food allergies, intense warning have to commonly be exercised. If you do have a meals allergic reaction, you may do your homework first. This can encompass making an appointment with the medical doctor or doing all of your private studies on the net, mainly on depended on clinical websites together with WebMD.

Allergy Remedy at Home

Are you allergic to some factor? If you do, you may be looking for places to get assist. While many humans inn to over-the-counter hypersensitivity treatment capsules or physician-prescribed hypersensitivity medicinal capsules, many others are inquisitive about getting to know extra approximately extra much less high-priced and herbal hypersensitivity consolation alternatives. If you're this sort of people, please hold reading due to the fact there are a few home remedies for masses precise varieties of allergies indexed underneath.

Before delving thru some domestic treatments which might be an wonderful and cheaper manner to gain help, it's miles essential to do not forget that clinic remedy is sometimes wished. For instance, if you have food allergies, you will be not able to use a enormous quantity of natural, home remedies because of the fact all of them require using meals. And, whether or not or no longer you revel in immoderate signs, collectively with issue breathing or loss of interest, it is essential which you searching out scientific hobby proper away.

Vitamin B5 is prescribed as a stable manner to ease allergic reaction signs and symptoms. It is well-known for presenting remedy to many allergic reaction sufferers. Vitamin B5 dietary supplements can and need to be taken on a ordinary foundation for at least a month. Others suggest using it on a everyday basis for an unspecified term, consisting of on the equal time as allergy court docket instances have appreciably reduced or aren't a trouble.

Another herbal and clean domestic hypersensitivity treatment is lime. To use this steady and home cure, squeeze the juice of one lime or half of of of a lime right into a lukewarm glass of water. If preferred, upload approximately a teaspoon of honey to this mixture. You must drink this lime mixture each day for some months. Many people go through in mind doing it first issue inside the morning. What's high-quality about this herbal hypersensitive reaction remedy is that it will also serve to detoxify the frame.

Bananas additionally can be used to spontaneously remedy allergies at home. For at least one month, one or bananas can be consumed on a normal basis. This solution is most amazing for all allergic reactions; however, those with meals allergies have to maintain with caution. In fact, bananas are not the most effective element that people with meals allergies can keep away from. Many which is probably allergic to three substances need to stop the use of natural remedies that comprise positive meals. Bananas, however, appear to advantage the ones who've pores and pores and skin reactions because of hypersensitive reactions the maximum.

In addition to the materials at the manner to benefit people with allergies, it is frequently beneficial to look at the meals and drinks that may be avoided. Allergy patients are cautioned to avoid caffeine drinks which encompass espresso and soda, in addition to beer. This is due to the truth that wonderful products include numerous additives. Additives cause the body to emerge as unnatural and impure. This isn't the way you need to be if you want to get allergy remedy.

The herbal treatments and home remedies for allergic reactions listed above are handiest a handful of the many who you can need to find out. Consider engaging in a preferred net quest for added answers which are handy, less high priced, and easy to contain at home. There are pretty numerous internet internet web sites available that offer unfastened get right of entry to to home treatments. Having said that, you'll probably despite the fact that need to spend money on home remedy books or publications tailor-made for allergy patients.

Where Do I Buy Allergy Medications?

Are you allergic to some aspect? If you do, you might be thinking about turning to treatment for help. If you are, you is probably thinking the manner to bypass approximately shopping allergy medicine. The proper records is which you have quite a few alternatives.

When it consists of choosing in which to buy hypersensitivity reliever tablets, it virtually is predicated upon on what you need or need to shop for. Prescription remedy, as an example, necessitates a clinical physician's be conscious. If, however, you choose to apply over-the-counter capsules, you will discover that you have a touch more leeway in phrases of purchasing opportunities. A few of the buying alternatives are said below.

As previously stated, pharmaceuticals for hypersensitive reactions have to need to be authorised via a scientific practitioner first. It is usually recommended which you make an appointment to get a prescribed drug. If you've got got have been given coverage, it is a first rate factor to get health recommendation and it's also plenty less pricey. If you've got coverage benefits, any form of prescription can be regular. If you do now not have drug coverage or if it's miles minimal, take a look at traditional manufacturers, which may be additionally masses a lot less high-priced. Simply go to one of the nearest pharmacies to get your prescription stuffed. If you've got coverage coverage, discover a pharmacy that offers it.

If you have got many pharmacies to choose from, you may undergo in mind numerous critical problems. Choosing the exceptional pharmacy is a exceptional deal extra vital than many humans apprehend. Choose a pharmacy that accepts the insurance, as formerly stated. Look for reasonably-priced fees as properly, as not genuinely everyone expenses the equal amount of cash. When you will pay a percentage extra than a well-known co-pay, or if you do no longer have drug blessings, store spherical. Customer care have to be scrutinized as well. Be high high-quality you have got had all your questions replied. You have to in no way depart a pharmacy with extra doubts than in advance than you arrived.

Like previously noted, with the resource of approach of purchasing over-the-counter hypersensitive reaction comfort medicinal tablets, you have were given have been given extra leeway. If you're involved about spending cash, one of the first locations you can skip is in your nearest department or dollar hold. These shops are well-known for his or her low prices. Having said that, they though sell call logo drug treatments, however at lower prices. Many off-marketplace or pharmacy logo medicinal pills are though available or for sale, which includes asthma reliever medicinal pills. Pharmacies may be found in loads of department stores, collectively with Wal-Mart, Kmart, and Target. This is useful if you need to are looking for advice from a pharmacist for the right over-the-counter hypersensitivity reliever medicinal pills.

Pharmacies are fantastic recognised for supplying prescribed drugs, but they also can offer the maximum over-the-counter gadgets. They also can have higher charges, however getting access to a big style of hypersensitivity drug treatments is a large benefit. While maximum hypersensitivity patients have quite some shopping selections, they sense greater comfortable whilst buying at a pharmacy or drug keep. It is likewise critical to emphasise the significance of preserving a pharmacist handy, mainly if you have any questions.

As handy as it's far to buy over-the-counter allergic reaction medicines locally, did you apprehend that you can even obtain this on line? You definitely will. There are some of online stores and supermarkets, which include Walgreen's and DrugStore.Com. For people who are constrained to their homes, searching the net for over-the-counter capsules is obtainable.

If you could see, there are some of picks to be had to you at the same time as looking for hypersensitivity remedy without the use of medication. To summarize, higher pharmaceuticals require a health practitioner's consent. Over-the-counter gadgets may be provided every on line and offline. To buy on line, behavior a regular internet search for the drug you want to buy. Visit the community department stores, eating places, consolation shops, and pharmacies for unbiased shopping.

Can Allergy Air Purifiers Really Work?

Are you allergic to some detail? If you do, you is probably continuously looking for techniques to remedy or manipulate your signs and symptoms and signs and symptoms. Despite the reality that there are numerous herbal and less costly alternatives to treatment hypersensitive reactions, some human beings are inquisitive about shopping hypersensitive reaction air purifiers. Most humans ask how air purifiers actually art work almost approximately hypersensitivity remedy before searching for one.

When it involves whether or no longer air purifiers can certainly cope with allergies, the bulk of the time, they do. In all fairness, it is counting on the form of air purifier used. Continue reading for greater detail approximately how air purifiers can be capable of provide you with allergy comfort, further to records about what form of air purifiers ought to be offered.

To understand how air purifiers can guide allergy patients, it's far necessary to first understand what they're. Air purifiers are transportable devices that easy the air. Their assignment is to dispose of pollutants from the air. Despite advances in technology, many air purifiers although rely on the usage of air filters. Many of the contaminants within the air could be trapped by means of manner of manner of those filters, preventing them from reentering.

Where it involves what kinds of contaminants are separated from the air, there are a few one-of-a-type particles which is probably accumulated and eliminated. Dirt, pollen, dirt mites, doggy threat, secondhand cigarette smoke, mould, and mold are all common air contaminants which can be eliminated. In terms of the way this may gain hypersensitivity sufferers, many have allergies to cigarette smoke, cats, pollen, mould, and mould. Many people will enjoy treatment as quickly as these items are removed from the air.

You may be interested by buying an air purifier and there can be a robust danger that it'll offer you with comfort from your hypersensitivity symptoms. If so, you is probably questioning which type of air cleaner is better. With such loads of air purifiers available in the marketplace nowadays, you could find out that you do have hundreds of selections. First, you may take a look at individuals who claim that permits you to assist with hypersensitive reactions. High-quit air purifiers and people that use HEPA air filters are greater expensive, however many people discover them to be properly well well worth the money.

You can also find out that you have a number of numerous alternatives even as it comes to shopping for an air purifier. Many customers like to shop for on-line. This is because of the gain and comfort of on line shopping, in addition to the capability to browse masses of stores with some mouse clicks. If you have not determined which kind of allergic reaction air purifier to shop for, you can want to begin via doing some on line have a look at. If you're looking for a few element locally, you may scope out your preferred home improvement stores.

As actual as it's far to recognize that an air purifier can be in a position to help you along with your allergic reaction signs, and as excellent as it is to recognize in which and the way to get them, it is also critical to recognize a manner to apply them properly. A complete-residence air purifier is prescribed for the excellent diploma of rest. If you can not have enough cash one, be selective on which rooms you located an air purifier in. Air purifiers ought to be utilized in areas which you use the maximum, which incorporates your take a look at, or in rooms wherein the hypersensitive reactions problem you the maximum. Make the maximum of your air cleanser, specially even as you're at home. If your air cleaner has an air clear out, make sure to clean or uninstall it as suitable.

To summarize, air purifiers act by means of getting rid of pollutants from the air, which incorporates dirt mites, mould, mildew, and doggy dander. When the use of an air purifier, hypersensitivity sufferers almost regularly are seeking out for a discount of their symptoms. Air purifiers are available for purchase each domestically and on-line.

How to Pick an Allergy-Relieving Air Purifier

If you need to eliminate the hypersensitivity signs and signs and symptoms and signs? If so, you can test air purifiers. Air purifiers are an first-rate way to alleviate most of the extra common hypersensitivity symptoms. In fact, a few people document that using an air purifier of their domestic surely gets rid in their hypersensitive reaction symptoms.

If that is your first time thinking about purchasing an air cleaner, you might be looking for recommendation. After all, there are masses of air purifiers within the marketplace proper now. If you sense annoyed with the aid of the use of all your choices, you may hold analyzing. For your ease, some buying guidelines for air purifiers are given under.

When searching out an air cleanser for hypersensitive reactions, it's miles recommended that you first examine HEPA air purifiers. HEPA-technology air purifiers are rather appeared and encouraged. Both air purifiers soak up and hold probable toxic particles from the air, such as mould, dust mites, and doggy dander, but a few are greater effective than others. On commonplace, HEPA air filters are stated to lure approximately ninety% of debris inside the air. This parent is a protracted way more than that of maximum tremendous air purifiers and air filters.

Another extremely good manner to discover a awesome air cleanser is to ask a person you meet for advice. You have to and can speak in your neighbours, colleagues, partner and youngsters, friends, and doctor. Air purifiers have grown in popularity in modern-day-day years. This is typically because of the reality that extra humans want to better their fitness and the air great of their homes. If you meet a person who makes use of an air cleanser, ask them for information about it. Do they like it? What are the blessings and drawbacks of proudly proudly owning?

Another advice for deciding on an air cleanser for allergy remedy is to do on line look at. If you need the price of an air purifier that you see available on the market close by, you may want to preserve off on buying it right now. Instead, make a have a study of the make and model and do your homework while you get home. Online, severa air purifiers are tested and checked. Reading comments and evaluating ratings will help you hold coins via eliminating air purifiers that aren't virtually genuinely worth the cash or are too expensive to govern.

It is crucial to undergo in thoughts consistency at the identical time as searching for an air purifier for allergic reaction treatment. As previously noted, ratings, feedback, and advice will assist you in determining the overall performance of an air cleanser. It's moreover well properly well worth noting that no longer all hypersensitivity air purifiers are made collectively, given that they yield severa outcomes. If you be afflicted by allergic reactions, you could want to locate the greatest viable comfort. Also, look for hypersensitive reaction-satisfactory air purifiers that consist of warranties. In contemporary, a assure suggests that a store certainly enables their devices, that would provide you with consolation and peace of thoughts.

When attempting to find an air purifier, go through in mind the rate as properly. It is usually critical to observe which you get what you pay for as regards to rate. High-surrender air purifiers are greater expensive, however most people deem them to be well clearly worth it. Try buying on line or at the least checking charges on-line first that will help you shop coins. It's also critical to bear in mind the lengthy-time period prices of proudly proudly owning an air cleaner. How an entire lot can filters get replaced once they will be used? How an lousy lot do they rate? When purchasing an air cleanser, preserve in thoughts that you may emerge as costing greater than the decal fee.

When attempting to buy an air cleaner, any of the aforementioned considerations have to be considered. As a reminder, now not all air purifiers are made collectively, so make certain you select out out the proper one.

What to Look for When Purchasing an Allergy Purifier

Are you allergic to a few aspect? If so, you'll be interested in purchasing an allergic reaction cleaner. Allergy purifiers are believed to lessen the quantity of signs and signs and symptoms skilled thru the use of the majority of hypersensitive reaction sufferers. If that is your first time thinking about shopping for an allergy air cleaner, you is probably uncertain about the way to hold.

When searching out to buy an allergic reaction purifier, it's far vital to understand that you do have a whole lot of buying options. This is important to understand as it will provide you with more companies to pick from even as nevertheless stopping you from overpaying. A few of your options for air cleaner searching for factors are said below.

It is also essential to remember that not all air purifiers are presented as "allergy purifiers." However, this does not suggest that they could now not reduce allergic signs. Mold, mold, dirt mites, secondhand cigarette smoke, and puppy dander are just a few of the probably toxic contaminants that maximum air purifiers clear out from the air. The absorption of those debris is what gives remedy to hypersensitive reaction sufferers.

As formerly cited, whilst seeking to purchase an hypersensitivity purifier, you have got an entire lot of alternatives. If you want to shop for regionally, you can visit your nearest home improvement shops. They frequently have the very tremendous kind of immoderate-prevent air purifiers in addition to the maximum vital choice of air purifiers. These immoderate-quit air purifiers are confirmed to last longer and offer superior typical performance.

Locally, you may even attempt out health shops, domestic development stores, and department stores. Since air purifiers are believed to increase the health of these stricken by hypersensitive reactions and allergic reactions, they will be regularly offered in fitness stores. Home and branch shops sell air purifiers as well, however the fact that their variety is generally constrained to decrease-surrender air purifiers which can be a good deal tons less luxurious to buy.

In addition to shopping for domestically, air purifiers can be sold at the net. When you operate the internet to do that, you may discover that you have pretty a few selections. As previously referred to, air purifiers are frequently bought in domestic improvement stores, home stores, scientific stores, and department shops. Many famous stores have on-line presences. You are welcome to go to the ones web web sites. Online, outlets ought to have a extra variety of objects, like purifiers, than they do of their brick-and-mortar locations.

As appealing as it's miles to do business enterprise with a acquainted save, you should no longer overlook smaller-scale operations, mainly those achieved on line. That is why you must behavior a regular internet experiment. You will use terms like "air purifiers available on the market," "hypersensitivity purifiers," or "allergic reaction air purifiers on the market" to accomplish that. A smooth internet are seeking for will lead you to on-line stores you couldn't have heard of in advance than. You can also be guided to an air cleaner manufacturer's on-line internet internet site online. If that is the case, you may be given a route to stores that sell their purifiers, or you could discover that a store has a web save wherein you may make your order right now from them.

Chapter 6: Review of Allergies

Your frame's reaction to in any other case slight fabric, along side pollen, mildew, animal dander, latex, nice substances, or insect stings, is referred to as an hypersensitivity. The signs and symptoms of an hypersensitivity might be moderate, collectively with a rash or hives, itching, a runny nose, or watery or crimson eyes, or they may be lethal. Antihistamines, decongestants, nasal steroids, hypersensitive reactions tablets, and immunotherapy are all sorts of treatment.

How do allergies art work?

Your frame system's reaction to a fabric it perceives as an dangerous "invader" is an hypersensitivity. For example, your immune machine, which serves as your body's protection mechanism, can also reply if it comes into contact with something in any other case hazard loose, like pollen. Allergens are the subjects that activate the ones responses.

An hypersensitive reaction is what?

Your frame's reaction to the allergen is called an "hypersensitivity." An allergy is the final consequences of a sequence of activities.

If you're at risk of allergies, your body will respond via developing hypersensitive reaction antibodies the number one time you are exposed to a specific allergen (which includes pollen). These antibodies are chargeable for finding the allergens and helping in their removal from your frame. Histamine is a substance that is secreted as a cease result and produces hypersensitivity signs and signs and symptoms.

Allergen kinds and treatment

You might probably have allergies to many diverse matters, together with pollen, animal dander, mold, and dirt mites.

Pollen

Hay fever, as well as seasonal allergic rhinitis, is an hypersensitivity to pollen. It inflames and swells the protective tissue during the eyes and the liner of the nose (conjunctiva).

Sneezing, stuffiness from congestion, and wet, scratchy eyes, nostril, and mouth are other symptoms and symptoms. Drinkable antihistamines, available with out a prescription and over-the-counter, anti-leukotrienes, nasal steroids, nasal antihistamines, and nasal cromolyn are some of the remedy possibilities. Pollen publicity in great men and women can result in the symptoms of allergic allergies (wheezing, shortness of breath, coughing, and/or tightness within the chest).

Avoiding pollen let you take away your symptoms. When pollen counts are immoderate, stay interior, near the home windows, and use the aircon. In order to remedy pollen allergic reaction, speak on your physician about immunotherapy (allergy injections).

Dust mites

Dust mites are little creatures which might be living inside the fibers of family objects which includes pillows, mattresses, carpets, and material in addition to in the dirt. Heat and humidity sell dirt mite boom.

Dust mite allergic reaction signs and signs and symptoms are similar to pollen hypersensitive reaction signs and symptoms and symptoms and signs and signs and symptoms. Use dirt mite encasements (hermetic plastic/polyurethane coverings) over pillows, mattresses, and box springs to help manipulate dirt mite allergies. Additionally, do away with the carpet or vacuum periodically using a excessive-efficiency filter out.

Care:

Medication may be used as part of your remedy to manipulate your chest and nasal/eye signs and symptoms and signs and symptoms. If avoidance techniques and remedy are inadequate to correctly manage your signs and symptoms and signs and symptoms and symptoms, immunotherapy may be counseled.

Molds

Molds are small fungi with spores that waft inside the air like pollen (like Penicillium). Allergies can end result from mould exposure. Mold can be placed outside inside the grass, leaf lots, hay, mulch, or below mushrooms and additionally indoors in moist regions similar to the basement, kitchen, or rest room. The amount of mildew spores will increase at some stage in the brand new season, and humid situations.

Care:

Medication may be used to deal with your chest and nasal/eye issues. If avoidance and medicinal drug are inadequate to sufficiently control your signs and symptoms, immunotherapy may be suggested.

A puppy's dander

Both the proteins in saliva and the dander released via using sweat glands in an animal's pores and skin have the capability to cause allergic responses. Avoidance works greater in comparison to clearly getting rid of the doggy from the residence. Second-great precautions, but, embody preserving your doggy out of your mattress room, making use of air cleaners with HEPA filtration, and regularly cleaning your pet (cat or canine), even though many people are unwilling to try this.

Care:

Medication may be used as part of your remedy to manipulate your chest and nasal/eye symptoms. If avoidance strategies and treatment are inadequate to effectively manage your signs, immunotherapy may be recommended.

Latex

After coming into contact with latex several times, some people get allergic to it. Rubber gloves applied in surgical operation or for family cleaning are a large contributor to this form of response. Symptoms of a latex hypersensitive reaction embody pores and pores and pores and skin rash, hives, eye watery and contamination, wheezing, and pores and pores and skin itching.

Latex hypersensitive reactions can reason minor signs and symptoms and signs and symptoms which consist of rashes and itching of the pores and skin. If your mucosal membranes are exposed, as they'll be after surgical procedure or a dental or gynecologic examination, greater excessive responses would in all likelihood appear.

Care:

Removal of the offending latex product is step one in treating latex reactions. It's important for human beings with latex hypersensitive reactions to place on Medic Alert® bracelets and supply emergency epinephrine kits each way.

Certain meals

When your frame creates a specific antibody in response to a high-quality meal, meals hypersensitive reactions are created. Within minutes after eating the item, an hypersensitive reaction occurs, and signs and symptoms might be very terrible. The most typical meals hypersensitive reactions in adults are to shellfish, peanuts, and tree nuts. Among these are milk, egg, soy, wheat, shellfish, peanuts, and tree nuts for kids.

Itching, hives, nausea, vomiting, diarrhea, breathing troubles, and swelling round your mouth are signs and signs of a meals allergy.

It is crucial to live faraway from food that get worse hypersensitivity symptoms. Your clinical medical doctor may moreover suggest you to usually bring injectable epinephrine (adrenaline) if you (or your infant) have a meals hypersensitive reaction. In case you via coincidence devour gadgets that purpose hypersensitive reactions, that is important. Oral immunotherapy is a unique treatment for peanut hypersensitive reactions.

Insect poison (stings)

A ordinary reaction to a bee stung includes pain, swelling, and redness at the edge net web site. Beyond the sting net internet site swelling is an indication of a severe community reaction. For example, in case you were stung on the ankle, your leg may also additionally growth.

An hypersensitive reaction to an insect sting is the most immoderate and requires rapid medical intervention. An allergy to an insect sting consists of the subsequent symptoms:

1. Breathing problems

2. Generalized (significant) hives—a purple, itchy rash that extends past the vicinity in which the bee turned into stung.

3. Facial, throat, or oral tissue swelling.

four. Wheezing or swallowing problems.

5. Anxiety and agitation.

6. Rapid heartbeat.

7. Lightheadedness or a surprising lower in blood strain.

A 2d sting might also moreover bring about a intense response that is probably lethal if you experience this form of reaction.

Care:

Epinephrine is a medication used to cope with allergies (adrenaline). If you have had a bee sting hypersensitivity, are searching out recommendation from a board-licensed hypersensitive reaction/immunologist to confirm your hypersensitive reaction with a pores and pores and skin and/or blood check. If venom hypersensitivity is diagnosed, venom immunotherapy is usually recommended. This will lessen the chance that a next sting may additionally result in a primary damage.

An allergic rhinitis definition

"Allergic rhinitis" is the time period used to explain hay fever and nasal allergy signs. Nasal allergies because of plant pollen that alternate with the seasons are known as seasonal allergic rhinitis (wooden, grasses, or weeds). Seasonal symptoms and symptoms take place sooner or later of a plant's pollination seasons. Your signs and symptoms can also moreover worsen at one in every of a kind instances of the yr or may be consistent because you may be allergic to many things.

Do everyone have allergic reactions?

No. The majority of allergies are hereditary, which means that that that dad and mom skip them at once to their offspring. Despite with out inheriting a selected hypersensitivity, people have a predisposition to be allergic. It is quite probable which you or your partner have allergies if your infant develops allergic reactions.

How commonplace is allergic reactions?

Allergies of every type, which include indoor/outdoor, meals, medication, latex, insect, pores and pores and skin, and eye allergies, have an effect on more than 50 million Americans (1 in 6). All age, sex, and racial lessons are seeing an growth in the quantity of human beings with allergic reactions.

Significance And Causes

What signs of allergies are there?

The severity of hypersensitive reaction symptoms can range from slight to severe:

Local symptoms and signs (signs and signs and signs and symptoms that handiest have an effect on one a part of your frame), which incorporates a rash or hives, itching, watery or red eyes, hay fever, and runny nostril, are examples of moderate responses. The consequences of slight responses do now not amplify to other bodily regions.

Symptoms that boom to specific regions of your body are indicative of a slight reaction. Itching, hives, swelling, and/or respiratory issues are possible signs and symptoms.

Anaphylaxis is an tremendous, life-threatening emergency in which your body's reaction to the allergen is abrupt and has an impact for the duration of your entire body. You may have intense facial or ocular infection in advance than anaphylaxis. Within mins, more excessive symptoms include throat swelling (which may additionally moreover make it hard to swallow and breathe), belly ache, cramping, vomiting, diarrhea, rashes, and swelling start to arise (angioedema). Due to the possibility of a blood pressure lower from anaphylaxis, you may additionally have highbrow disorientation or dizziness.

Why do allergies occur?

An hypersensitivity may be brought on through the use of some factor you come into contact with that your body perceives as a "volatile intruder." Common allergens encompass pollen, animal dander, mold, dust, additives, insect venom, and latex, all of which may be frequently harmless objects.

Technically talking, a series of actions taken via way of your body in reaction to the "negative intruder" are what reason your signs and symptoms. Your body "sees" the intruder, produces antibodies to combat it, and as a cease end result, histamines that motive allergic symptoms are launched.

Tests And Diagnosis

How is an allergic reaction analysis made?

Do no longer wait to appearance whether or not or not or no longer your symptoms and signs and symptoms go away if you suspect that you have allergic reactions. Make an appointment with an allergy/immunology expert in case your signs and symptoms persist for greater than per week or two and in all likelihood to head again.

The allergens inflicting your allergy signs and symptoms and symptoms and signs and symptoms can be positioned through hypersensitivity pores and skin trying out. The test includes pricking your pores and skin with an allergen extract and seeing how your pores and pores and skin responds.

Blood checks can be used if a pores and skin test is not possible. As against a pores and pores and skin take a look at, this one is a whole lot less touchy. The take a look at measures what number of antibodies your immune tool produces. A probably allergy to that allergen is typically endorsed by way of way of higher degrees of fantastic antibodies.

There are more hypersensitivity attempting out options to be had.

Control And Treatment

How is the remedy for hypersensitive reactions?

Although warding off the allergen is a important part of remedy, the allergic response commonly might no longer surrender absolutely.

Your allergy signs and symptoms and symptoms and signs and symptoms are treated with pills like antihistamines (e.G., Allegra®, Zyrtec®), decongestants (e.G., Sudafed®, Contact®), or a mixture of over-the-counter and pharmaceuticals. Cromolyn sodium, topical nasal antihistamines, and topical nasal steroids like Flonase® and Nasonex® can all be used as nasal sprays to treat allergy symptoms.

The following bronchial allergies tablets reduce hypersensitive reaction symptoms:

- Inhaled bronchodilators.

- Inhaled steroids.

- Oral bronchodilators.

- Oral anti-leukotrienes (montelukast, zafirlukast and zileuton).

- Injections, which includes omalizumab , dupilumab , reslizumab , benralizumab , or Mepolizumab.

Chapter 7: The perfect natural (natural) remedy for hypersensitive reactions

Avoidance is the super natural treatment for allergic reactions while it's far realistic. Allergens, which are what triggers your hypersensitive reaction, should be confined or avoided, regular with each scientific professionals and alternative healers.

You have to preserve your allergies at bay. For example, inform your doctor in case you've ever skilled an negative reaction to a sulfa remedy. If you ever need an possibility antibiotic, they'll possibly prescribe one.

However, a few hypersensitive reactions is probably hard to avoid. In such example, after speaking together together together with your clinical clinical medical doctor about your symptoms, you can don't forget the usage of a home cure for hypersensitive reactions to cope with the consequences of being exposed to an allergen.

Home remedy for allergic reactions

Nasal irrigation with saline

The outcomes of 10 research showed that saline nasal irrigation become effective for treating allergic rhinitis, or hay fever, in every kids and adults.

Air purifiers

In your interior environment, don't forget the use of an air clean out.

One type of air smooth out to recall is a HEPA smooth out (immoderate-efficiency particulate air). The amount of allergens in your own home is decreased through way of HEPA filters, which seize airborne irritants along aspect pollen, dirt, and puppy dander.

Butterbur

It modified into decided that butterbur, additionally called Petasites hybridus, works clearly as nicely for indignant eyes as a normal traditional antihistamine.

Bromelain

An enzyme known as bromelain can be positioned in papaya and pineapple. Natural healers consider that bromelain is useful for reinforcing respiration by means of reducing edema.

Acupuncture

Additionally, studies show that acupuncture is powerful for treating allergic rhinitis, each seasonal and perennial.

Probiotics

23 researches from a Reliable Source encouraged that probiotics can also assist with allergic rhinitis signs.

Honey

A notably common notion recommends consuming regionally produced honey, but the lack of scientific evidence to useful resource it. The hypothesis states that over the years, you will become lots a lot much less allergic to the pollen that bees acquire for your vicinity to manufacture their honey.

Air conditioners and dehumidifiers

Air conditioners and dehumidifiers can lessen the formation of mildew and mold, that may have a harmful influence on allergies, via removing moisture from the air.

Spirulina

Additionally, nutritional spirulina, a shape of blue-inexperienced algae, has been proven to have anti-allergic defensive homes in competition to allergic rhinitis.

Injurious nettle

Stinging nettle is typically encouraged thru the usage of practitioners of opportunity treatment as a herbal antihistamine to resource inside the treatment of allergic reactions.

Quercetin

Natural treatment proponents encompass quercetin because of the truth they think it stabilizes histamine release and decreases allergy signs and signs. It occurs truly in meals which consist of citrus quit end result, inexperienced tea, broccoli, and cauliflower.

Vitamin C

Natural medicinal drug experts endorse eating 2,000 mg of weight-reduction plan C each day to lower histamine stages.

Peppermint oil, critical

According to a 1998 assessment, the usage of peppermint oil to treat bronchial allergies and allergic rhinitis signs and symptoms and symptoms faded their severity enough to useful resource medical research. Although they may be used topically, crucial oils want to be diluted in a issuer oil in advance than being subtle into the air.

Eucalyptus oil, essential

During hypersensitivity season, proponents of herbal treatment endorse which includes eucalyptus oil to each cycle of laundry as an antibacterial agent.

Frankincense oil is used.

According to the findings of a 2016 test, frankincense oil may be effective in treating continual allergic rhinitis. You can diffuse it into the air or examine it at the back of your ears after diluting it in issuer oil.

Possible Precautions while the use of domestic remedies for hypersensitive reactions

Avoid using herbal treatments to deal with anaphylaxis, a excessive allergic reaction that could consist of signs and symptoms like:

Difficulty breathing

Lung constriction

Chest ache

Alterations in blood stress

Dizziness

Fainting

Rash

Vomiting

Seek short scientific help in case you expand those signs and symptoms. Anaphylaxis poses a excessive risk to lifestyles.

Additionally, the usage of critical oils consists of a few risk. The purity, first-rate, and packaging of critical oils are not underneath the control of the U.S. Food and Drug Administration. Use of critical oils is crucial as to make certain you're using awesome items as cautioned.

On unbroken pores and pores and skin, together with your forearm, check the crucial oil diluted in provider oil. It have to be good enough to use if you do no longer respond to it inside 24 hours. Test each new vital oil in advance than the usage of it, in particular if you have hypersensitive reactions. And in chapter seven of this e-book, we are able to study some of the beneficial and extensively applied requirements.

Chapter 8: Seasonal Allergies: Signs, Diagnosis, and Therapy

Hay fever is a term most usually used to seek advice from seasonal allergic rhinitis (an hypersensitivity). It affects 8% of Americans, on common.

Your immune machine overreacts to an outdoor allergen like pollen, which motives hay fever. What reasons an allergic reaction is called an allergen. Pollens from wind-pollinated plants, which includes weeds, grasses, and bushes, are the most not unusual allergic reactions. Pollen from plant life which are pollinated with the beneficial resource of bugs is sincerely too heavy to stay within the air for terribly prolonged and is lots a lot much less in all likelihood to purpose an hypersensitive reaction.

The word "hay fever" refers back to the time of 12 months whilst hay is reduce. In the beyond, this interest came about inside the direction of the summer season, around the time that many human beings started out to boom symptoms.

Although seasonal allergic reactions are a splendid deal less frequent in the wintry climate, allergic rhinitis can stand up at any time of the one year. At severa intervals of the yr, many flowers launch their very personal pollens. You can also moreover want to undergo hay fever in a few unspecified time in the future of a couple of season, relying on your allergic reaction triggers and the climate wherein you live. Additionally, indoor allergens like mould or cat dander would possibly cause a response in you.

Seasonal allergic reaction symptoms and signs and symptoms

Seasonal hypersensitive reactions can motive moderate to immoderate symptoms.

The most common ones are:

Sneezing

Runny or congested nostril

Itchy and watery eyes

Sinuses, throat, or ear canal itchiness

Congested ears

Drainage from the nose

Less common symptoms embody:

Headache

Breathing issue

Wheezing

Coughing

Asthma impacts a massive type of hay fever sufferers. Seasonal allergens also can motive an allergic reactions assault if you have hay fever and allergic reactions.

Seasonal allergy triggers

Your immune system errors a usually consistent airborne chemical for a hazard, resulting in hay fever. Histamines and different chemical substances are released into your device in reaction to that substance, or allergen. These substances reason allergy signs.

Seasonal variations have an impact on what often gadgets off hay fever.

Spring

The majority of seasonal allergic reactions in spring are as a result of spring wood. In northern latitudes, wherein many people with hay fever respond to its pollen, birch is one of the worst offenders. Cedar, alder, horse chestnut, willow, and poplar are a number of the opposite allergenic wooden determined in North America.

Summer

The summer season months are generally on the equal time as hay is lessen, therefore the moniker "summer season hay fever." But ryegrass and timothy grass, similarly to several weeds, are the primary motives of seasonal allergic reactions in the summer time. Grass is the maximum not unusual allergen for those with hay fever, consistent with the Asthma and Allergy Foundation of America.

Fall

Ragweed season is in the fall. Ambrosia is the genus name for ragweed, and there are extra than forty species of it in the course of the sector. The majority of them flourish in North and South America's temperate climates. They are difficult to manipulate invasive flora. Their pollen is a surprisingly commonplace allergen, and ragweed allergies may have very bad signs and signs and symptoms.

Nettles, mugworts, sorrels, fats hens, and plantains are among one of a kind flowers that launch pollen within the fall.

Winter

The majority of outdoor allergens are dormant via wintry weather. As a quit result, many hay fever sufferers find out respite in bloodless climate. However, it moreover way that greater humans are staying interior. If you are prone to seasonal allergic reactions, indoor allergens like mold, domestic dog dander, and dust also can purpose you to moreover experience signs.

It is from time to time much much less tough to get rid of indoor allergens out of your environment than outside pollens. Here are a few tips for placing off common hypersensitive reactions in your own home:

• At least as quickly as each week, wash your bedding in extremely heat water.

• Use coverings which can be proof in opposition to allergens in your pillows and beds.

• Get rid of upholstered furniture and carpeting.

• Take filled animals out of your kids' bedrooms.

• Address water leaks and remediate water harm to prevent the boom of insects and mould.

• Wipe off any moldy regions and capacity breeding grounds, at the side of humidifiers, swamp coolers, air conditioners, and freezers.

• To take away more moisture, use a dehumidifier.

Diagnosing of seasonal hypersensitive reactions

Compared to one of a kind allergens, hay fever is normally simpler to diagnose. If you're allergic reactions quality appear in the path of specific seasons of the year, you could have seasonal hypersensitivity rhinitis if that is the case. In order to make a diagnosis, your medical doctor should furthermore observe your throat, nose, and ears.

Typically, allergic reaction trying out isn't required. No remember what shape of allergen you're sensitive to, your treatment for allergic rhinitis will possibly be the same.

Seasonal hypersensitivity treatment

The notable treatment for allergic rhinitis and hay fever is to stay far from the allergens that make you feel sick. Additionally, there are medicinal drugs for hay fever symptoms. Others check with complementary treatments.

Avoidance

Be proactive approximately warding off seasonal hypersensitive reactions. For instance, within the summer, opt for an air conditioner with a HEPA filter over ceiling fans to relax your private home. For pollen forecasts, take a look at your neighborhood climate network, and try to live interior at the same time as there are plenty of pollens. When your hay fever is energetic at a few degree inside the 12 months:

• Keep the windows closed.

• Limit it sluggish spent out of doors.

• When you are outdoor, specially on windy days, think about the usage of a dirt masks.

Additionally, smoking need to be averted due to the fact it might make hay fever signs and symptoms and signs and symptoms worse.

Medication

Other treatment options are to be had in case you aren't capable of avoid your allergic reactions, including:

• Over-the-counter pills comprising acetaminophen, diphenhydramine, and phenylephrine in addition to decongestants and antihistamines such cetirizine.

- Prescription pills, together with nasal steroid sprays

If the signs are intense, your doctor must suggest hypersensitivity injections. They are a shape of immunotherapy which could beneficial useful resource in decreasing your immune device's sensitivity to allergens.

Some hypersensitivity capsules may have undesirable factor effects like disorientation, sleepiness, and dizziness.

Chapter 9: What Leads to Seasonal Allergies?

One kind of allergic reaction is allergic rhinitis. It takes place whilst some thing for your environment triggers an excessive immunological reaction.

In precise terms, your frame responds to a reason from the surroundings that is frequently secure as although it have been a deadly disease or some extraordinary sort of danger.

The signs and symptoms of allergic rhinitis frequently resemble cold signs and symptoms and signs. For example, they'll be:

Sneezing

Runny or congested nose

Wet or itchy eyes

Coughing

Headache fatigue

You probable have an indoor reason allergic reaction if you have it all one year round. Discover the maximum today's indoor allergens that purpose allergic rhinitis all 12 months prolonged.

Pet dander

Tiny fragments of animal pores and skin which have died and fallen off make up dander. It is gift within the surroundings and on devices that come into contact with animals.

Dander adheres to apparel, furniture, and carpet with out issues when you remember that it is minute, slight, and has tough edges. As a stop stop end result, it spreads fast in a region, like your home

Pet dander may also cause hypersensitivity responses, but top notch sorts are greater vulnerable to do so than others. For instance, the American Lung Association estimates that cat hypersensitive reactions are approximately two times greater common than dog hypersensitive reactions.

Additionally, no longer all dog breeds are suitable for hypersensitivity patients.

It's feasible that some "hypoallergenic" canine breeds have a decrease chance of causing an allergy.

Poodles and schnauzers are some of the canine with non-dropping coats that the American Kennel Club (AKC) recommends as extra steady breeds for hypersensitivity patients.

Tips

Consult your health practitioner in case you need a doggy but are sensitive to domestic canine dander. Find out in the event that they assume you'll be greater stable with precise animals or kinds.

If you currently possess a puppy, take motion to lessen the amount of dander in your home. For example:

• Regularly deliver your puppy a tub.

• Regularly vacuum each the furniture and the floors.

• Wash and replace your bedding often.

• Refrain from letting your domestic dog indoors your mattress room or on any furniture.

• If you've got were given carpet, consider removing it, or not less than, frequently vacuum and smooth carpet and rugs.

Mold

A form of fungus called mildew flourishes in moist environments. If the proper events are met, it could increase almost anywhere. For example, it frequently develops round or on:

•   Walls and flooring in lavatories

•   Basements, garages, and sheds

•   Air conditioners

- Refrigerators

You're much more likely to experience mildew troubles if your private home has terrible air waft and excessive humidity tiers.

Tips:

Advice on preventing the development of mildew

Place lovers in moist areas. Use the bathroom exhaust fanatics, as an example, even as taking a shower.

In regions that experience humid or scent musty, set up a dehumidifier. Make tremendous you routinely smooth the dehumidifier's coils and filters.

Get rid of any property of greater moisture. For instance, recuperation roofs or pipes which is probably dripping.

Keep your home's drainage structures, which includes gutters, clean.

If mildew takes over a space in your own home this is greater than 10 rectangular ft, you may need to don't forget hiring a expert to easy it up.

Dust mites

Tiny insects called dust mites are living in domestic dust. They consume every airborne moisture and pores and skin cells from people. The dirt is also made up of their our our our bodies, saliva, and excrement, which might in all likelihood reason an hypersensitive reaction.

Tips:

Advice for keeping off dirt mites:

Cover your pillows and mattresses with plastic zipped coverings.

Wash all your location rugs and bedding in warm water on a ordinary foundation.

Tile or timber flooring should take the place of carpet in your house.

Instead of curtains, use hard window coverings like blinds.

Vacuum your home often. Invest in a vacuum with a excessive-performance particulate air (HEPA) filter out, after which frequently smooth or replace it in line with the manufacturer's instructions.

Cockroaches

Several bugs, collectively with cockroaches mainly, can reason allergic responses.

You can inhale cockroach excrement, saliva, and microscopic frame additives, just like each different allergy reason, if they may be discovered in your own home or place of work.

It is extensively recognized that cockroaches are resilient and difficult to put off. They can live on in almost any surroundings, no matter the reality that they select locations wherein there may be sufficient of moisture and food to be determined.

Tips:

Advice for heading off an infestation:

Never leave pup or human food out.

Cover your rubbish packing containers, wash your dishes, and take away any food crumbs proper away.

Your partitions and floors also can have cracks which you need to seal to save you cockroaches from getting into.

Sources of greater moisture have to be regular or wiped smooth up.

Use baits and traps to kill cockroaches.

Regularly have an exterminator spray.

Prevention

Avoiding your triggers is a important component of controlling your hypersensitive reaction symptoms if you have allergic rhinitis.

Consult your medical doctor in case you're uncertain of what is causing your allergic reactions. They are in a function to suggest an allergist to test you. When you have got decided what is inflicting your signs and symptoms and signs and signs and symptoms, you could take precautions to prevent it.

By preserving a clean and nicely-maintained house, you could lessen the amount of indoor allergic reaction triggers. For instance, frequently update your bedding and vacuum your floors, fixtures, and cloth.

Your ability to reduce the amount of indoor allergy triggers is likewise advanced with the aid of using fixing leaks and other belongings of greater moisture.

Chapter 10: Allergies to pollen

What is an hypersensitivity to pollen?

To fertilize particular plants of the equal species, wooden, flowers, grasses, and weeds generate pollen, a very great powder. Additionally, it's miles most of the maximum famous causes of allergic reactions inside the u . S . A ..

When they breathe in pollen, many human beings revel in poor immunological reactions.

Normally, the immune device protects the frame in opposition to illness-causing invaders like viruses and bacteria.

When someone has a pollen allergy, their immune device misinterprets hazard free pollen as a possibly unstable invader. To fight the pollen, the immune tool begins to create materials like histamine.

The actual shape of pollen that reasons it's far referred to as an allergen, and this is known as an allergic response. Numerous bothersome signs, which encompass sneezing, a stuffy nostril, and watery eyes, are delivered on thru the hypersensitive reaction.

Some humans have hypersensitivity symptoms all three hundred and sixty five days spherical, at the same time as others simplest accomplish that now and again. For example, folks which might be allergic to birch pollen commonly revel in worsening symptoms and signs within the springtime, at the same time as birch trees are in blossom. Similar to this, the early fall is the worst time for humans with ragweed allergies.

An individual's pollen allergy is not going to head away as soon as it has manifested. However, medicines and allergic reaction injections may be used to alleviate symptoms. Additionally, some manner of life adjustments might possibly useful resource with symptom remedy.

ARE YOU AWARE? Hay fever or seasonal allergic rhinitis is exclusive names for a pollen allergic reaction.

In 2018, 7.7% of adults and 7.2% of children in the United States had hay fever, in step with the Centers for Disease Control and Prevention's National Health Interview.

Types of hypersensitive reactions to pollen

There are numerous plant species that produce pollen and purpose allergic responses in people.

Some everyday offenders embody:

- Tree birch

- An very welltree

- Grass Ragweed vegetation

Birch pollen sensitivity

One of the most normal hypersensitive reactions within the springtime is birch pollen. Tiny pollen grains are launched as birch wooden blossom, and the wind disperses them.

5.Five million Pollen grains can be produced thru the usage of a single birch tree.

Oak pollen hypersensitive reaction

In the spring alrighttrees like birch wooden launch pollen into the atmosphere.

Compared to the pollen of numerous wooden, okaypollen is concept to be most effective slightly allergic, but it remains inside the air for an prolonged amount of time. Some human beings who are touchy to pollen may additionally get excessive allergic responses due to this.

Pollen allergic reaction to grass

During the spring and summer time, grass is the primary deliver of pollen hypersensitive reactions.

There are numerous types of grass. Only a small style of flora, on the side of perennial rye, Bermuda grass, and bluegrass, can motive allergic reactions.

Allergies to ragweed pollen

The weeds that are maximum at risk of motive allergies are ragweed vegetation. Nearly 1 billion pollen grains can be produced by using way of one plant.

They are busiest in the first few weeks of autumn. However, ragweed can start dispersing its pollen as early as August and maintain doing so until November, depending at the region.

The wind-borne pollen also can bear a slight wintry weather and excursion loads of kilometers.

Allergic signs and signs to pollen

Most regularly, pollen hypersensitivity symptoms consist of:

Nasal clogging

Sinus pressure can also result in face ache.

- Clogged nostril

- Wet, itchy eyes

- Unwell throat

- Cough

- Blue, swollen pores and skin in the back of the eyes

- Reduced potential to taste or fragrance

- Increased responses to allergic reactions

Pollen allergy reasons

When your immune device interprets pollen as a probable unstable fabric, pollen allergies growth.

Any sort of hypersensitivity, which includes a pollen hypersensitive reaction, has an unknown etiology. According to specialists, genetics might be involved.

Pollen allergy analysis

A pollen allergic reaction also can furthermore frequently be identified via a number one care health practitioner. To confirm the prognosis, they might deliver you to an allergist for hypersensitivity testing. An expert in figuring out and treating hypersensitive reactions is called an allergist.

These actions are normally involved in allergic reaction finding out:

Step 1: Your clinical facts and cutting-edge-day signs and symptoms is probably mentioned, which encompass when they first appeared, how long they've got lasted, and if they're ordinary or trade over the yr.

Step 2: To end up aware of the incredible allergen causing your signs and symptoms, they'll next behavior a pores and skin prick test. They will puncture numerous factors of the pores and pores and skin at a few degree in the technique and inject a touch quantity of certain allergens.

Step three: Within 15 to twenty minutes, the area will become purple, swollen, and itchy in case you are allergic to any of the components. Additionally, a raised, round location that resembles hives can be seen.

Allergy remedy for pollen

Despite taking precautions, if symptoms persist there are remedies that might be useful.

Medications

There are numerous over-the-counter (OTC) allergic reaction drug treatments, along with:

Antihistamines like Cetirizine and Diphenhydramine (Benadryl) Decongestants like Pseudoephedrine and Oxymetazoline Combination medicinal pills like

Loratadine/Pseudoephedrine and Fexofenadine/Pseudoephedrine.

Allergy injections

Allergy pics may be encouraged in case your symptoms and symptoms can not be managed by using the use of drug treatments.

Shots for allergic reactions are one example of immunotherapy. The allergen is injected normally into you. Over time, the allergen interest inside the injection progressively rises.

Your immune device's reactivity to the allergen is altered via the injections, which permits reduce the intensity of your allergic responses. The American Academy of Allergy, Asthma, and Immunology states that after taking hypersensitivity injections for a year, you could attain tremendous treatment. A enormous of 3 to 5 years of remedy may be required.

Immunization in competition to allergic reactions isn't always endorsed for kids below the age of 5.

Home remedies for allergic reactions to pollen

Several natural remedies can also be used to address pollen hypersensitive reaction symptoms and signs and symptoms and signs.

These encompass:

• Flushing pollen out of the nostril with a squeeze bottle or internet pot.

• Trying herbs and extracts like spirulina or PA-loose butterbur (which do not encompass risky pyrrolizidine alkaloids).

• Removing and cleaning any outside-worn clothes.

• Using a dryer to dry clothes in region of a clothesline outdoor.

• Making use of air con in houses and motors.

• Making a buy of a dehumidifier or portable excessive-typical overall performance particulate air (HEPA) clean out.

• Using a HEPA-filtered vacuum purifier on a normal foundation.

How to keep away from hypersensitive reactions to pollen

As with specific hypersensitive reactions, warding off the allergen is the high-quality technique to save you signs and symptoms of a pollen allergy.

But it might be hard to keep away from pollen. Nevertheless, you might be capable of lessen your pollen publicity with the aid of:

• spending dry, windy days interior.

• Delegating outside or gardening chores to others in some unspecified time in the future of busy times.

• Donning a dirt mask at some point of periods of excessive pollen counts.

• Securing domestic home windows and doorways sooner or later of periods of immoderate pollen ranges.

Chapter 11: Allergies to ragweed

What Is an Allergy to Ragweed?

United States is domestic to ragweed plant life, that have sensitive stems. The ragweed that grows in North America is certainly one of at the least 17 wonderful species. Rural settings and large locations with masses of mild are in which the plant life are most regularly placed. Ragweed vegetation produce little pollen grains inside the direction of the past due spring and fall months to fertilize extraordinary ragweed plant life.

Ragweed can start dispersing its pollen as early because the final week of July and hold till the middle of October, relying at the region. Its wind-borne pollen can also undergo a mild wintry weather and excursion hundreds of kilometres.

One of the most conventional triggers of seasonal allergies within the US is ragweed pollen. When they breathe within the pollen, many humans enjoy detrimental immunological reactions. In order to prevent infections, the immune machine commonly protects the body from risky intruders like viruses and bacteria.

Ragweed pollen is misidentified as a hazardous chemical through manner of the immune system in sufferers with ragweed hypersensitive reactions. Despite the pollen being harmless, this triggers the immune machine to create molecules that combat toward the pollen. Numerous grating symptoms and signs and symptoms and signs and symptoms, which includes sneezing, runny nose, and itchy eyes, are brought on by using the reaction.

A ragweed allergic reaction influences round 26% of Americans. Once an allergic reaction has manifested, it's far now not going to move away. However, drug treatments and hypersensitive reaction injections can be used to relieve symptoms and signs and symptoms and symptoms. Changing some elements of 1's way of life can also assist reduce the outcomes of ragweed hypersensitive reactions.

What Allergic Reactions to Ragweed Are There?

Depending on wherein you stay and the weather, your signs and symptoms and signs and symptoms might also additionally trade at a few level inside the 12 months. But the most contemporary ragweed allergy signs and symptoms and symptoms and symptoms and symptoms are as follows:

☐   Wet, itchy eyes

☐   Throat soreness

☐   Congestion or a runny nose

☐   Wheezing or coughing Sinus pressure can also result in facial pain

☐   Bluish-coloured pores and skin in the back of the eyes this is swollen

☐   Reduced notion of taste or scent

☐   Poor notable of sleep

Some those who are uncovered to ragweed pollen also can furthermore have allergic eczema. This slight, itchy rash regularly consists of tiny bumps and blisters. Within 24 to 48 hours of exposure, it is able to show up. Usually, the rash will go away on its private in to 3 weeks.

Other irritants, in conjunction with cigarette smoke, powerful scents, or air pollutants, would possibly possibly exacerbate signs and symptoms. The Environmental Protection Agency claims that ragweed allergies may be getting worse because of climate trade. A longer pollen season for ragweed can also additionally end result from warmer temperatures. They might also additionally stimulate ragweed to generate more pollen.

What Leads to an Allergy to Ragweed?

When the immune tool reacts improperly to ragweed pollen, a ragweed allergic reaction develops. Normally, the immune tool encourages physiological adjustments that resource in the frame's protection in competition to volatile invaders like germs and viruses. But in humans with ragweed allergies, the immune tool misinterprets the innocent pollen as a adversarial invader and starts to war it. The frame reacts to ragweed pollen thru freeing chemical referred to as histamine. Numerous unpleasant signs introduced on with the useful resource of the histamine consist of runny nose, sneezing, and itchy eyes.

Ragweed is a member of the Compositae family of flowering plant life. These plants may be located in all 50 states, several locations in Canada, and temperate South American areas. Ragweed pollen is specifically difficult to keep away from for the motive that it can be inhaled via someone and then come into contact with them. The peak month for ragweed pollen manufacturing is September, and the season normally lasts from August via mid-October. . Around 10 a.M., pollen levels are frequently at their most. Depending at the weather, among three p.M. Pollen levels can be decreased with the beneficial resource of rain and bloodless climate.

Ragweed pollen hypersensitive reactions are extra acquainted within the ones who have hypersensitive reactions to exclusive chemical substances. If you have got hypersensitive reactions to any of the subsequent, you're more likely to develop ragweed hypersensitive reactions:

Dust mites

Mold

Pet hair

Various pollens, together with tree pollen

Since allergies additionally frequently run in families, you're much more likely to grow to be allergic to ragweed if a member of your instantaneous own family does.

How is an Allergy to Ragweed Diagnosed?

A ragweed allergy can also commonly be identified through your professional. To verify the diagnosis, they will ship you to an allergist for allergy checking out. An expert in identifying and treating hypersensitive reactions is referred to as an allergist. Your scientific history and present day-day signs and symptoms and signs, which include after they started out and how lengthy they have got lasted, is probably cited with the allergist first. Tell them whether or not or no longer the symptoms and symptoms and signs excellent appear or worsen at unique periods of the year.

After that, the allergist will do a pores and pores and pores and skin prick check to discover the proper allergen causing your signs and symptoms. The normal skin prick technique is as follows:

The allergist makes use of a pen or marker to mark a part of your arm or returned.

Then they take a look at droplets of numerous allergens to numerous pores and pores and skin-touch elements.

The skin locations wherein those drips are present are softly poked or scraped with a needle. It can be a bit unsightly or painful, but it in reality takes a few minutes to complete.

Within 15 to twenty mins, the location turns into red, swollen, and itchy in case you are allergic to any of the substances. Another feasible sight is an improved, spherical region that resembles a beehive.

You and the allergist will speak the findings. You have to have allergies to severa different things.

A pores and pores and pores and skin prick take a look at give up quit result may not usually advise that you are allergic to the drug. The findings of the pores and pores and skin prick test and the allergist's non-public medical assessment may be used to make a evaluation and develop a treatment approach.

How is an Allergy to Ragweed Treated?

Because ragweed pollen is so difficult to avoid, you can probable maintain to have allergic responses. However, there are some of medicinal tablets that might ease the signs and signs and symptoms of ragweed allergies.

Medications

The following medicinal drugs can reduce signs and symptoms:

Antihistamines together with diphenhydramine or loratadine

Decongestants like oxymetazoline and pseudoephedrine Nasal corticosteroids which include mometasone and fluticasone.

Drugs like Actifed and Claritin-D that mix an antihistamine with a decongestant

If over-the-counter medicinal pills do no longer art work, communicate for your doctor approximately prescription drugs. The prescription treatment montelukast should quality be taken if there aren't any special powerful treatment options to be had because of the danger of immoderate negative consequences.

Allergy images

If pharmaceuticals aren't supporting, your health practitioner should endorse allergic reaction injections. A collection of injections of the allergen is utilized in hypersensitivity images, a shape of immunotherapy. Over time, the allergen recognition inside the injection often rises. Your frame's reactivity to the allergen is altered thru the injections, which allows lessen the intensity of your allergic responses. After starting allergic reaction injections, you could have standard treatment interior one to three years.

There are one of a kind sublingual immunotherapies to be had to cope with ragweed allergies. In this form of therapy, a tablet containing the allergen is swallowed after being placed beneath the tongue. It offers similar blessings to hypersensitive reaction injections.

Personal Changes

Additionally, you can regulate your way of life to lessen your threat of developing ragweed allergic reactions:

•   Use an air conditioner in some unspecified time within the future of the summer season and into the autumn.

•   When pollen ranges are at their top in the morning, keep away from going outdoor.

• Purchase a transportable dehumidifier or immoderate-efficiency particulate air (HEPA) clean out.

• Use a vacuum with a HEPA smooth out to smooth the house as soon as in line with week.

• After wearing garb out of doors, wash it proper away to put off any viable pollen.

• Instead of drying your garments outside on a line, use a dryer.

Foods to exclude

Some ingredients and plants may moreover motive an allergy due to the reality they encompass proteins which can be similar to those placed in ragweed pollen. These consist of:

• Bananas

• Chamomile

• Cantaloupes

- Cucumbers

- Echinacea

- Melon honeydews

- Watermelon

- Zucchini

Typically, the season of ragweed will make food hypersensitive reaction signs and symptoms worse. If you revel in tongue tingling or itching after consuming any of the aforementioned devices, you need to consult an allergist.

Chapter 12: Aromatherapy (Essential Oils) for Allergies

Seasonal hypersensitive reactions may additionally strike inside the overdue wintry weather, early spring, or perhaps the late summer time and early fall. Occasionally, hypersensitive reactions might in all likelihood seem even as a plant to which you are allergic blossoms. Or, in some unspecified time in the future of particular seasonal months, you can have regular allergic reactions.

The signs and symptoms of hypersensitive reactions can be handled alternatively or moreover the usage of essential oils. They come from plants and characteristic a vast style of programs. Typical applications for crucial oils encompass:

• Airborne diffusion of them.

• Making use of them in spa and tub goods.

• Using them on the pores and skin after diluting them.

• Dispersing them in the ecosystem.

• Taking breaths of them without delay from the container.

Aromatherapy is the act of respiration in the fragrances of essential oils. Your frame is stimulated via the usage of using this interest via heady scent. Your body's extraordinary structures may be impacted via what you smell.

Applying the oils to your body reasons them to go into your bloodstream, similar to with aromatherapy. Before using critical oils to your pores and skin, you need to always dilute them.

For this, issuer oils like sweet almond oil or olive oil may be powerful. Typically, five drops of the important oil are used to as a minimum one ounce of service oil.

There isn't plenty of data to again up the usage of essential oils, but new research are constantly being published. You must gain from aromatherapy in case you workout it cautiously.

Here are some important oils you'll probably need to strive in case you need to use them to your existence to lessen allergic reaction symptoms and signs and symptoms.

1. Lavender

Due of its many blessings, lavender vital oil is a famous desire.

Its capacity to loosen up and reduce irritation also can assist you control your symptoms within the route of allergic reaction season. According to at least one test, the important oil stops allergic contamination and the increase of mucous cells.

Diffuse lavender for aromatherapy talents or lighten up in a bathtub of diluted lavender oil.

2. A combination of Ravensara, Frankincense, and Sandalwood oil

In one studies, chronic allergic rhinitis have become treated with a aggregate of sandalwood, frankincense, and Ravensara oils. The clogged nasal passageways, runny and itchy noses, and sneezing of look at individuals all progressed.

This manner that this aggregate of crucial oils may be capable of decorate said symptoms, allergy-associated great of existence, and sleep.

Apply the ones mixed oils to the face after combining with a service oil (which consist of candy almond oil). They can also be dispersed in the environment.

three. Eucalyptus

Since eucalyptus oil is an anti-inflammatory, it is able to relieve your congestion. As you deal with and manage seasonal hypersensitive reactions, the chilling sensation you get even as respiratory it in may also provide some consolation.

The mechanism thru which eucalyptus aromatherapy lowers inflammation is beginning to grow to be easy to researchers. This should bring about a lower in hypersensitivity symptoms.

Eucalyptus oil can be inhaled instantly from the container or subtle into the air for relaxation.

Despite having anti inflammatory developments, some humans's hypersensitive reactions is probably aggravated via eucalyptus.

Chapter 13: Comparing sulfa and sulfite hypersensitive reactions

Sulfonamide allergies, regularly known as sulfa treatment allergic reactions, are instead general.

In the Thirties, sulfa medicinal capsules proved to be the primary effective treatment for bacterial ailments. Antibiotics and other drugs, which includes diuretics and anticonvulsants, retain to comprise them. Sulfa sensitivity is particularly risky for those who've HIV.

People frequently mistake sulfa for sulfites because of their names being similar. Most wines actually include sulfites. They are also utilized in particular meals as preservatives. Despite having no chemical connection, sulfites and sulfa drugs can each make humans touchy to them.

Allergy to sulfur

An allergic response to sulfa includes the subsequent signs and signs:

• Hives

• Face, mouth, tongue, and throat swelling

• Blood pressure decline

• Anaphylaxis (a intense, life threatening reaction that calls for on the spot medical attention)

Rarely, responses same to serum contamination could likely happen 10 days after beginning a sulfa treatment treatment. These signs and symptoms include:

• A fever Skin rashes

• Drug-introduced on arthritis, hives

• Enlarged lymph nodes

If you've got any of these symptoms, you want to peer a medical doctor right away.

Drugs to persuade clean of

If you've got sensitivity to sulfa or are allergic to it, stay far from the following tablets:

Antibiotic combination medicines encompass trimethoprim-sulfamethoxazole, erythromycin-sulfisoxazole, sulfasalazine, that's used to cope with Crohn's illness, ulcerative colitis, and rheumatoid arthritis, and dapsone, it is used to

Safe capsules for those who've sulfa allergic reactions

Sulfonamide-containing medicinal tablets do now not geared up off responses in every person. The following pills can be efficaciously utilized by many humans with sulfa hypersensitive reactions and sensitivities, even though they have to be desirous about caution:

a.   Several diabetic tablets, which include glimepiride and glyburide.

b.   Medicine for migraines sumatriptan.

c.   Several diuretics, which embody furosemide and hydrochlorothiazide.

It relies upon on the person whether or not or no longer they could take those meds or now not. Consult your clinical physician when you have a sulfa allergy and are dubious when you have to take any of these drugs.

Chapter 14: Special Advice

Call a doctor

Inform your health practitioner if your signs get worse or if the factor outcomes that your allergic reaction pills are causing grow to be bothersome.

Additionally, get clinical advice in advance than utilising any novel herbs or dietary supplements. Some can avoid a remedy's functionality to art work well.

Consult your medical physician

If you trust you studied you'll be allergic to sulfa or sulfite, see your medical physician to installation the outstanding course of movement. You may additionally want to have extra checks or are seeking out recommendation from an expert. If you've got were given bronchial allergies specially, make certain to speak approximately collectively collectively along with your medical doctor the medication and devices you need to stay far from.

Chapter 15: Know Your Enemy

The best way to combat your allergic reactions is to first pinpoint the motive of them. Are they environmental, puppy associated, food associated or seasonal? Prior to trying any answer, you want to find out this difficulty, or these elements and then decide whether or no longer it is for your energy to dispose of yourself from the out of doors state of affairs or when you have to address the difficulty via outdoor solutions. When figuring out your hassle, it is important to first decide your hypersensitive reaction, and differentiate most of the motive, outdoor factors and the reactions.

For instance, pollen can be the purpose of many human beings's hypersensitive reactions. Since it is frequently seasonally decided, the seasonal prevalence may be the outdoor factor. Lastly, the consequences of the pollen at the body which incorporates runny nose, watery

177

eyes, or itchiness might be the allergies. All of these mitigations play a big element in helping you discover the treatment that you want.

This financial disaster records some of the pinnacle reasons and locations of vital allergies, a prerequisite to discovering the notable solutions for you.

Allergy Type 1: Food

For many people, tremendous foods can cause slight, slight or intense allergies. If you have got got have been given this type of allergic reactions, they will be extra tough to combat apart from outright avoidance. However, for your comfort underneath are listed the most common food hypersensitive reactions. In the united states, the beneath substances make up ninety% of meals associated allergic reactions.

1.Peanuts

2.Tree nuts

three.Milk

4.Eggs

five.Wheat

6.Soy

7.Fish

eight.Shellfish

Allergy Type 2: Environmental

Believe it or now not, in which you live can play a primary function for your publicity to allergens and thereby boom your chance of probabilities for unfavourable reactions. Below are states with the very pleasant large form of pollen consistent with the Asthma and Allergy Foundation of America.

Worst locations to live for allergies:

1. Louisville, KY

2. Memphis, TN

3. Baton Rouge, LA

four. Oklahoma City, OK

5. Jackson, MS

6. Chattanooga, TN

7. Dallas, TX

eight. Richmond, VA

9. Birmingham, AL

10. McAllen, TX

Allergy Type three: Pets

Despite their cuddly trends and potential to wiggle their manner into our hearts, a few pets can reason a few essential hypersensitive reactions. The primary purpose for doggy allergies are the hypersensitive reaction inflicting elements located of their fur or dander. So, in case you seem to like animals however no longer your hypersensitive reactions, beneath are some of the most famous hypoallergenic pets accessible.

Best pets for allergic reaction inclined animal enthusiasts:

1.Portuguese water canine

2.Sphynx cat

three.Kerry blue terrier

4.Standard Poodle

five.Devon rex cat

6.Bichon fries

7.American Labradoodle

8.Syrian hamster

9.Leopard gecko

10.   Goldfish

Allergy Type four: Popular Allergen Triggers

For many human beings, a commonplace allergen is pollen. However, there are a huge variety of similar triggers available that people do now not even understand they're being constantly exposed to. Below are some of the maximum not unusual.

1.Pollen- Known to trigger hay fever, seasonal allergies, and a plethora of other signs (ie. Runny nose, itchiness, red eyes), pollen is common in maximum environments and can be incredibly hard to keep away from making it one of the primary reasons of allergies in human beings.

2.Mold- Not only can it harm the indoors of homes however moreover it can further harm you via the use of the usage of triggering unwanted hypersensitive reactions. Spores of this fungi go with the go along with the waft round in the air inflicting your signs. Since they're in substantial decided in damp regions which includes toilets or basements it may be tough for plenty to avoid. Prevention is typically the splendid mode of treatment for this. Keep your house easy and dry to prevent its prevalence.

three.Dust Mites- These tiny, dust living organisms may be hard to keep away from. Prevention may be the important component proper right here. Since they will be now not particular to fine seasons you have got were given got the threat of being constantly exposed to them, so, if possible, cover any surfaces dust mites are regarded to are living and generally wash material collectively with bed sheets and garments with warmth water to rid them of any of those organisms and one in every of a kind allergens.

Allergy Type five: The Rest of the World

Keep in mind that the above commands had been certainly some of the maximum not unusual. The scope of allergens isn't always limited to the aforementioned types. So, if your allergies do no longer flawlessly align with them, do now not try to motive them to in shape. While the ebook gives herbal remedies to some of these common issues, strive now not to definitely rule out the choice of speaking to a clinical professional. Your private physician and close by medical doctor may be treasured resources close to your warfare in competition to pesky allergies.

www.ingramcontent.com/pod-product-compliance
Lightning Source LLC
Chambersburg PA
CBHW062138020426
42335CB00013B/1252